PRAISE FOR *MOM, UNFILTERED*

"Courageously written; cathartic and healing to read. Kim invites readers into some of the most devastating, unspoken experiences of motherhood with candor, vulnerability, and hope. Through her personal story and socio-political analyses, Kim makes an irrefutable case for how our society fails mothers while drawing us a map to collective healing and home."
—**Bianca Mabute-Louie**, author of *Unassimilable: An Asian Diasporic Manifesto for the 21st Century*

"*Mom, Unfiltered* is medicine for these times. It is a call for honesty, repair, and collective care. Leah Kim gives voice to realities of motherhood that are often kept secret, makes meaning out of suffering, and offers a way through to healing. By weaving her own story with the experiences and wisdom of other mothers, she has created a tapestry of truths that will set us all free."
—**Layla F. Saad**, *New York Times* bestselling author of *Me and White Supremacy: Combat Racism, Change the World, and Become a Good Ancestor*

"Leah Kim is a change agent who writes like someone trying to remake the world in the image of progress. Her sentences don't just imagine change; they insist on it. Until the reader, too, begins to believe in the possible."
—**Frederick Joseph**, *New York Times* bestselling author of *Patriarchy Blues: Reflections of Manhood* and *This Thing of Ours*

"*Mom, Unfiltered* is essential reading not just for mothers and birthing people but also for their partners, loved ones, and caregivers. Leah Kim's book is nothing short of revolutionary."
—**Poppy Liu**, actress, activist, mother, and doula

"*Mom, Unfiltered* level-sets the playing field for parents, guardians, coparents, and social justice warriors alike by crystallizing what this moment needs: collective care, love, and community."
—**Joél Leon**, author of the 2025 Gotham Book Prize-nominated *Everything and Nothing at Once: A Black Man's Reimagined Soundtrack for the Future*

"*Mom, Unfiltered* is such a refreshing and honest look at motherhood. Leah Kim isn't afraid to tackle the tough stuff—racism in healthcare, generational trauma, and mental health—while reminding us to hold on to faith and grace through it all."

—**Anita Kopacz**, bestselling author of *Shallow Waters*

"Leah Kim's brilliant vulnerability in *Mom, Unfiltered* gently unravels the shame woven into motherhood without losing sight of the systems that distort our path. She makes space for our imperfections, shares her own inherited trauma and generational patterns, and pulls no punches, calling out capitalism, racism, and white supremacy. I laughed out loud, teared up more than once, and finished feeling held by this beautiful confessional. It reminds us of our precious humanity and the divine right to evolve."

—**Ashley Simpo**, writer, doula, and mom

"While motherhood is so often publicly championed, Kim takes us through the gritty reality: it remains under-resourced and misunderstood, especially for the marginalized. In *Mom, Unfiltered*, she unravels the myths that abound, removing old dressing, bringing new gauze and needed air. Through soaring memoir and sobering research and history, Kim points us toward a liberated and joyful renewal of the role of mother and all the ways we need each other through its arduous labor, birth, and on. I am moved by her harrowing and heartrending work that has opened me repeatedly to a better vision of support, as the role of parenting requires all of us and more of us."

—**J.S. Park**, BCC, hospital chaplain and author of *As Long As You Need: Permission to Grieve*

"*Mom, Unfiltered* is the radical motherhood narrative that we all need for our collective healing. All humans, regardless of whether or not they ever choose to give birth or raise a child, would benefit from reading this book."

—**Yumi Sakugawa**, author of *There is No Right Way to Meditate*

"*Mom, Unfiltered* is an essential read for every young woman navigating life and identity in America. With raw honesty and lyrical grace, it captures the universal journey of motherhood, both its vulnerability and its quiet triumphs. More than a story, it's a fearless self-investigation that balances emotional depth, heartbreak, and healing in equal measure."

—**Naley by Nature**

Mom, Unfiltered

Maternal Mental Health and Finding Freedom Through Motherhood

Leah Kim

BLOOMSBURY ACADEMIC
NEW YORK • LONDON • OXFORD • NEW DELHI • SYDNEY

BLOOMSBURY ACADEMIC
Bloomsbury Publishing Inc, 1359 Broadway, New York, NY 10018, USA
Bloomsbury Publishing Plc, 50 Bedford Square, London, WC1B 3DP, UK
Bloomsbury Publishing Ireland, 29 Earlsfort Terrace, Dublin 2, D02 AY28, Ireland

BLOOMSBURY, BLOOMSBURY ACADEMIC and the Diana logo are trademarks of
Bloomsbury Publishing Plc

First published in the United States of America 2026

Library of Congress Cataloging-in-Publication Data
Names: Kim, Leah author
Title: Mom, unfiltered : maternal mental health and
finding freedom through Motherhood / Leah Kim.
Description: New York : Bloomsbury Academic, 2026. |
Includes bibliographical references and index.
Identifiers: LCCN 2025030797 (print) | LCCN 2025030798 (ebook) |
ISBN 9798881842437 hardback | ISBN 9798881848965 pdf |
ISBN 9798881848958 epub
Subjects: LCSH: Kim, Leah | Maternal health services | Postnatal care |
Postpartum depression | Mothers—Mental health | Minority women—Mental health
Classification: LCC RG940 .K575 2026 (print) | LCC RG940 (ebook)
LC record available at https://lccn.loc.gov/2025030797
LC ebook record available at https://lccn.loc.gov/2025030798

ISBN: HB: 979-8-8818-4243-7
ePDF: 979-8-8818-4896-5
eBook: 979-8-8818-4895-8

Typeset by Deanta Global Publishing Services, Chennai, India
Printed and bound in the United States of America

For product safety related questions contact productsafety@bloomsbury.com.

To find out more about our authors and books visit www.bloomsbury.com and sign up for
our newsletters.

Contents

Introduction

I saw a sign once. It said: "Be the person you needed." I think about this often.

I have been a mother for just over a decade now. My kids are six and a half years apart. We didn't expect to have a second child because my first postpartum period was so terrifyingly bad. I sometimes still can't believe we all made it through.

I think of my firstborn, my son, as my warrior partner. His birth brought out the darkest—and strongest—parts of myself. I have also been my worst self in front of him, unconsciously acting out what was done to me as a child. This has been incredibly painful.

As a longtime yoga practitioner and teacher, by the time I was first pregnant, I thought I had my life and my mental health under control. I understood my body, I meditated, I ate well. I was the picture of health.

When my son was born, I was in the middle of what would be a ten-year contract with Nike as their first-ever global yoga ambassador. I underestimated the pressure I felt to have a particular kind of birth story, to get my body back, and to essentially erase all evidence of having become a completely new person.

For the longest time, I thought that this was just a me-problem, that I had failed myself, that I was failing as a mother. But in the countless conversations I have had with other mothers—whether their children are newborns or fully grown adults who are now parents themselves—I have come to realize that many if not most mothers struggle, because there simply are no systems to support us.

I wrote *Mom, Unfiltered* to illuminate the myriad ways that society systemically fails all mothers with a particular focus on the challenges for mothers with marginalized identities. *Mom, Unfiltered* braids my own foray into motherhood with analytical examinations of privilege, accessibility, generational and lived trauma, racism, capitalism, colonialism, and more. It speaks to an experience of motherhood much more inclusive than the dominant conversation.

Over ten chapters, I'll cover various aspects and stages of motherhood and provide relevant cultural context, testimonies from mothers of various backgrounds, research, and expert insight. The most common picture of motherhood that we are sold is incomplete at best, a blatant lie at worst, absent of the reality of overwhelm, isolation, anxiety, and disconnection that many mothers feel. Through my personal stories of traumatic birth and insufficient maternal care, I'll illustrate specifically the damaging impact that the systemic marginalization of people of color has on a mother's mental health.

I'll also explore American diet culture, the white beauty standard, the capitalist project of the momfluencer economy, and the white, American tendency against community and how these social forces intersect with motherhood, often causing suffering that can manifest as mental or physical illness. Further still, I'll dissect the yoga world's white-led focus on toxic positivity and spiritual bypassing and how it hampers effective and necessary mental health care, particularly for mothers with BIPOC and immigrant identities who are prone to experiencing lived and generational trauma which can include abuse. BIPOC mothers, like me, are already tasked with raising BIPOC / biracial children in a world rooted in white supremacy, adding yet another layer of challenge to our mothering. Mothers urgently need support and while therapy can be life-changing, it can be either inaccessible or unhelpful if devoid of cultural competence.

Each of these themes is central to my personal experience, and throughout the book I will be brutally honest, vulnerable, and revealing—from agonizing over my own inherited rage issues to deeply transparent conversations about obsessive dieting. I'll also show how these struggles and oppressive systems actually impact *all* mothers, irrespective of racial identity. Through medical statistics, social research, and expert interviews we will see that these issues are all deeply intertwined and systemic. Ultimately, we confront the harsh realities of a hostile world.

This book is, however, hardly pessimistic—in fact, it's deeply hopeful. This is a book of survival and growth, an invitation for mutual support and a look at moving through trauma, abuse, and discrimination to create a kinder and gentler existence on the other side.

Mom, Unfiltered is most urgent for the mother who is feeling disconnected from herself and her family. She may or may not have an official diagnosis of a postpartum mood disorder—or she may feel alone in her community. This book is for the mother who feels unseen, underrepresented, and oppressed, especially those with BIPOC, immigrant, and all other marginalized identities. This book is for the mother without her own mother and without a village. The mother who has no model of motherhood to rely on, whether in the flesh or in memory. The mother who has experienced childhood trauma. The mother feeling voiceless and uncared for.

Throughout the book, I interchangeably use the terms mother and birthing person. I honor each person's chosen identity. I invite all of us to accept each other exactly as we are. I believe our own healing and liberation start there.

A mother's mental health matters because it impacts her ability to mother. It impacts her children, who are the ones inheriting this beautiful, but hurting, world. When a mother heals, her children heal, her own inner child heals, her ancestors heal, and the collective heals. This work is sacred.

I wrote *Mom, Unfiltered* to be the person I needed in my darkest days, in the hopes that I might also be able to bring light to another mother who is currently trying to find her way out of darkness.

May we all know that we are not alone.

1

Birth

My birth plan for my first child was as follows.

My birth partner would be my husband, Giles.

I would give birth in a pool at the birthing center. That was the more *natural* option, of course. How nature intended us to give birth. In fact, what I really wished for was being in a forest near a river, plopping into Malasana—a yoga squat pose—and the baby simply sliding out thanks to gravity and how good of a yogi I was.

I am a realistic person, though, so a birthing pool would be just fine, and luckily, the hospital I was zoned for in East London—Homerton Hospital—had a birthing center that was connected to the main hospital. Best of both worlds, just in case . . . not that a just-in-case scenario could ever possibly be relevant for me.

I wanted absolutely no intervention. No medicine—not even laughing gas. I was a yogi—a yoga teacher! I would obviously simply breathe through all of it.

My placenta encapsulist would be waiting to receive my placenta, so I would need that ready for her immediately. We would come prepared with a large, sterilized Tupperware box, ice packs, and a keep cool bag. Skin-to-skin as soon as possible, no bottles or pacifiers (because nipple confusion!), and we want to be discharged as soon as possible.

We had taken exactly two hypnobirthing classes so we were obviously totally ready.

Whenever I talked about my birth plan with anyone, I was so confident and assured. I knew I could manifest the perfect circumstances for the perfect birth. I never even considered *What If* scenarios; I dare not let the word *cesarian* even enter my consciousness. If I didn't think it, it couldn't happen.

The period leading up to your due date is pretty wild. There you are, expecting what is the biggest arrival and change and responsibility to your very existence but you have no idea what's going to happen. You don't know what kind of experience you're going to get or how you're going to get it. You really have no control in any of it, but it's all happening in your own literal body. It's a mindfuck, albeit a sacred one.

The due date itself is but a best estimate. It can even be edited as your pregnancy progresses in the early weeks, based on the growth rate of your baby. But none of it is exact because humans are not factory-produced robots. We are miracles of cells joining and dividing and dividing again.

According to the American College of Obstetricians and Gynecologists, "Only about 1 in 20 women give birth on their due dates."[1] So when my water broke on my due date, I took it as a sign that everything was going to go to plan.

I messaged two of my girlfriends, one of whom had just had a baby and the other who was imminently expecting her second.

"I guess he's coming today after all! My water broke and the mucus plug came out!" I texted.

"OMG! Where's Giles?"

"He's at work." I answered casually.

"Is he on his way home to take you to the hospital?"

"You mean *birthing center*," I corrected my friend. "No, I haven't told him yet. I haven't felt any contractions."

"But your water definitely broke?"

"Yes."

"Call Giles, and go! The baby is coming!"

We arrived at the hospital and I was quickly sent to an examination room where they confirmed that my waters were indeed gone.

"Waters, plural?" I asked, wondering if I had heard wrong.

"That's right. Both the front and back waters broke."

"Is that . . . bad?"

"No, dear, it's what is supposed to happen. It usually happens because of contractions, but 1 in 20 women do have waters breaking before contractions. Don't worry, they will likely start soon and you will know when they do! But for now, go home and rest. You'll probably be back later today. At the latest, make sure to return 24 hours from now, even if contractions haven't started."

Somehow through all my planning and preparation, I had not considered the possibility of contractions never starting. It must not have happened to any of my friends, because I had never heard about this. According to the National Health Service, England's health-care system known as the NHS, "The length of time between your waters breaking and contractions starting varies. We can't predict on an individual basis how long it may be but we know that about 6 in 10 (60%) women will start labor naturally within 24 hours."[2]

Naturally.

That had to be me. I lived to be *natural.*

So we went home, holding all the layers of feelings knowing that we would be holding our son the next day.

The following morning was bright blue sunny skies—not the most common for the Old Smoke. I wonder if I will ever forget walking into the hospital, clutching my pillow from home, painfully naïve to what lay ahead. I see this memory as if I had always been outside of it, watching myself from above, bidding farewell to the person I used to be, a person that didn't know they were about to all but disappear.

Contractions still had not started which was 40 percent to be expected. I wasn't worried and I didn't sense any urgency from any of the hospital staff.

The hospital was more crowded than usual, they said, and so I was given a bed in the post-cesarian ward (an omen, in hindsight). I was periodically checked and except for some traces of meconium, which I guess was normal, I was told everything was fine.

Eleven hours and zero contractions later, I was finally taken into a delivery room and put on Pitocin to induce labor. This was the next most natural option, rather than rushing to other interventions. I was disappointed how off track my birth plan I was getting, but there were still things I could insist on.

Refusing the epidural was one of these things.

The midwife said, "Darling, are you sure? The contractions that come on from induction tend to be more erratic and more intense. Most women opt for pain relief."

Bouncing on the yoga ball, I answered, "Yes, I'm sure. But I actually have a pretty good pain tolerance. If I change my mind later, I can always get the epidural then, right?"

"You technically can, but you may need to wait. There are only two anesthetists on staff and they are always very busy and may not be able to get to you right away."

"I see. Well, I feel fine now, so, I'll just wait."

"Are you sure, dear?"

"I'm sure!" I said cheerfully, insisting on manifesting a narrative where I could heroically claim that I did not have an epidural. Whose hero was I trying to be anyway?

I had a TENS machine, bought over the counter at my local pharmacy, which some people swore by for pain relief. The NHS *says* that "TENS—transcutaneous electrical nerve stimulation—is a treatment that gives temporary pain relief. A TENS machine passes a weak electrical current to your nerves which can help ease pain." A weak current providing temporary pain relief—I was sure that would be sufficient.

The midwife came back to check on me four hours after I was put on the Pitocin drip. Contractions had finally started, and they were feeling totally manageable. I declined the epidural again (was my birth plan not right there for everyone to refer to??) and I carried on with my yoga ball bouncing and gentle stretching.

I'm not sure exactly when the blinding pain started but in recounting it with my husband, I think it was at about the five-hour mark. The pain went from manageable in one instant to indescribable in the next. It felt like a bus, or a bull, was trying to ram its way out of my vagina. I was in such pain that I was rendered mostly mute, except to meekly ask the midwife if I might please be able to have that epidural now?

She ran to call for an anesthetist but as she had warned me, neither was available in that moment. One passed by my door and I remember him peeking in and saying, "I am so sorry, I have to go to emergency surgery. I will come back for you as soon as I can."

For two hours, I (pointlessly?) pressed the buttons on the TENS machine. I writhed in pain. At one point, I looked up and through my long black hair that had become matted to my face with my tears and my sweat, I saw maybe four or five midwives and nurses around me.

"This poor girl."

"Is the anesthetist available yet?"

"Hang on, sweetheart, relief is coming."

"Can somebody call for the doctor?"

Finally, the anesthetist was back. I swear when he entered the room, he was surrounded with golden sparkly beams of light. He was an angel, a savior. He got right to work, talking me through the procedure as he was setting everything up. I signed the paper agreeing to the risk. He told me I had to try my very best to be as still as possible so he could insert the needle in the exact right spot in my spine. I felt an icy cold.

And just like, the pain vanished. I whispered, "Thank you so much," slowly moved from the fetal position onto my back, and fell asleep.

Over the next ten hours or so, we continued to wait. At a certain point, they had to attach a fetal heart monitor to my baby's head. He has always, still, had a bald spot there. He was starting to show some signs of distress, but I was told that we were not in an emergency situation just yet. I desperately wanted the opportunity to be able to push, to birth my son *naturally*.

Birth in the UK is midwife-led. If you have no complications, you won't see a doctor, not even once. Even at this point, I had only seen a doctor very briefly, when I was first put on Pitocin.

My heart sank when I saw that he was back at my bedside.

Another doctor, a woman, was with him this time, because they were just upon shift change. They both explained to me that although I was fully dilated, things were not progressing as they would like. The baby was okay, but they didn't want to keep him in there any longer.

My options were to go into surgery now, to try manual intervention, or to wait one more four-hour cycle before going into surgery.

The truth was, I rejected all of these options. Why was this happening? What had I done wrong? I had eaten well and exercised throughout my entire pregnancy. I taught yoga up until a few days before my due date. I was one of the healthiest people that I knew. I could accept not getting to deliver in a pool but please, God, at least let me deliver without surgery! I had never once had any surgery except for getting my wisdom teeth pulled, if that even counts.

The manual intervention failed, but I think it must have been then that they realized he was twisted at the neck and stuck in the birth canal. They pushed to go to the operating theatre, as they call it in the UK, but I begged for more time.

I remember seeing Giles in his favorite denim shirt, on the other side of the room. He was bouncing on the yoga ball now, mustering enthusiasm and cheering, "Let's go, you can do this, let's go for one more cycle!" I know he, too, was manifesting not needing to go to surgery because he was worried about me and because he just wanted both the baby and me to be safe. But part of me wondered if he would be disappointed if I needed surgery. Would he think I had failed?

And then it all happened in the blink of an eye.

"Baby's in distress. Call the consultant to meet us in theatre."

"Leah, we're moving you to theatre now, it's time to get this baby out. Now."

Did I say anything in response? Did I nod? Did I consent? Would it have mattered? Did I at least put on a brave face?

There were so many people now. I was put onto a steel table. The anesthetist was staying with *me* now, I was the emergency surgery now. I will never forget his kindness, his calm. He was never out of my eyesight. The epidural was at maximum now. Was my body still there? I couldn't feel anything. I could only turn my head from one side to the other.

My teeth were violently chattering.

"I'm cold," I whispered.

More blankets were placed on me. Giles was told to sit next to the left side of my head. He was told to stay on *this* side of the blue curtain that was put up. To shield us from the upcoming splicing of seven layers of skin, the removal of my organs in order to retrieve our baby.

They would give me one last shot at a vaginal delivery with the aid of forceps. It would require me to push, to push harder than I had ever pushed with my vagina. Had I ever pushed with my vagina?

I couldn't feel anything.

I tried. I tried to push. I really tried.

I failed.

I looked at the clock. 12:00 p.m.

My teeth chattered.

I'm sure I must have prayed.

At 12:20 p.m., we finally heard the cry. He was here. He was okay.

I couldn't see anything that wasn't in my direct periphery so I looked at Giles who was looking for his first born. His son. Our son.

"Is he okay?" I asked, over and over again.

He was placed in Giles' arms.

"Oh he's so cute!" I cooed. Not because I could really see him or take anything in yet, but because that's what a mother is supposed to say.

Giles didn't look happy. I searched his face, trying to understand his expression.

Was our baby okay?

"Uh, excuse me?" he called out to someone, anyone. "Is he okay? His head looks . . . kind of squashed? And this one eye, uh, doesn't seem to be opening?"

We were told that the indentations on his head were to be expected after the forceps, but that they would eventually go away. And that it was normal that he was still figuring out how to open his eyes.

The epidural was slowly wearing off. Did I properly convey my gratitude to the anesthetist? I was eventually propped off the operating table and back onto the hospital bed, this new human being, my little guy placed in my arms. Although he ended up being not so little at nearly nine pounds, which was probably why he got stuck inside my apparently narrow birth canal.

But it was all good. He was here. We were both alive. Everything was going to be okay.

* * *

Giles went out to get us food. I started messaging loved ones: "Whew, giving birth is crazy! But we made it!"

I urged Giles to go and sleep at home that night. By then, it would be our third consecutive night in the hospital and I wanted him to go and check on our puppy. (Oh, by the way, did I mention we had gotten a puppy when I was eight months pregnant?) I had the midwives and nurses to help me; the baby and I would be fine.

Except that we weren't.

In the middle of that first night, something alarmed the nurses. Maybe it was the intensity of the baby's cries, I'm not sure—there's so much I don't fully recall. Two doctors appeared at my bedside once again. They took my baby from me and when they returned, they did not bring my baby back. They needed to run tests, they said, by way of a lumbar puncture. They slowly informed me that this procedure carried the risk of paralysis.

"Paralysis?" I asked, completely dumbfounded. But I had gone through three and a half days of labor and everything was fine. He was fine. Wasn't he?

"It's very unlikely to happen, but we do need you to understand that it is a risk. It's also the only way we can know what is going on and how to treat him."

"Who will be doing the lumbar puncture?"

"I will," one of the doctors answered.

"Have you ever . . . paralyzed a baby?" I could not believe we were having this conversation, less than twenty-four hours after my baby had been born.

"No, I have not."

"Has it happened here in this hospital before?"

"Yes, it has."

When I try to make sense of my postpartum darkness—which for me included diagnoses of depression, anxiety, panic disorder, and PTSD—my brain brings me to this moment. This was the moment when I went into a self-protective mode. An involuntary numbing. I envision a stone wall being erected around my heart.

How else could I shield myself from the possibility of my baby being paralyzed?

I called Giles. I remember his voice sounding so far away. We were both stoic, detached, exhausted. Shock, probably.

"Okay, if that's what the doctors are saying we need to do, then I guess we need to do it," I heard him say.

I signed a paper, like I had ahead of the epidural, again acknowledging risk and promising not to hold the hospital responsible.

I waited with bated breath to hear how the puncture had gone. One of the doctors returned to inform me that it unfortunately, had not worked. It's a blind jab, he explained, and they hadn't been able to obtain any spinal fluid. So they had to do another one. Another blind jab into my baby's spine.

I am sure I must have prayed.

They eventually brought him back to me, not paralyzed, thank God, just with a giant bandage that nearly covered his entire tiny back. He was crying more ferociously than before. Of course he was! He had just been poked with needles and he was not even one day old! I struggled to hold my worry.

We ended up staying at the hospital for a total of eleven days. We watched so many other families come and go. We waited for answers. Giles chased down one doctor after another.

Was our baby okay?

What was wrong with him?

Did the tests come back yet?

Was it meningitis like the doctors feared, or not?

Our baby had to go to NICU but because the post-cesarian ward was next to the NICU, after the first day, they allowed us to wheel him in and out for his medicines and tests.

Everything felt out of control.

Nothing had gone to plan.

I took my first shower and gritted my teeth in pain and fear, grateful for the rails attached to the walls, not knowing how to best protect my still-open wound. I wanted to go outside and breathe fresh air but I was told I was not allowed to leave the ward as long as my baby was still admitted.

Breastfeeding felt impossible. My milk took even longer to come in than it does for most mothers, which can happen with a traumatic birth. I insisted on trying to EBF—exclusively breastfeed—even as my son was hungry, irritable, and losing weight. I just couldn't bear to *poison* him with formula. Formula was not natural.

One night, in the desperation of exhaustion and confusion over how to soothe my baby, I called for a midwife. She came in and expertly picked up my baby. I looked on, helpless and afraid.

"He won't stop crying."

"This baby's hungry," she said, with a deep, experienced certainty. I was trying, I told her, but he wouldn't feed. She offered to make him a bottle, and panic gripped me.

"Won't it cause nipple confusion? I have to be able to breastfeed my baby."

"There is no such thing as nipple confusion. All these crazy things they tell you poor mothers to scare you. Your baby is hungry. He needs to eat," she said.

What about his brain development? All the bad stuff I had heard about? She calmly told me she had mix-fed her own babies.

"They are all grown up now," she told me. "There is absolutely nothing wrong with their brains."

I agreed to a bottle and I watched in amazement as the midwife deftly held, soothed, and fed my newborn. He guzzled that bottle in seconds.

"Ah," she whispered, "You see? He's hungry."

She made him another bottle. He finished it.

I was grateful and relieved in the moment but still, I did not want to formula feed my baby.

There were posters all over the hospital ward warning against using pacifiers, or as the English inexplicably call them, dummies. I was being brainwashed about "breast being best," but why? For whose benefit and at whose detriment was this insistent messaging?

It felt like I was being set up for failure at all the turns. There was a clear winning birth narrative that indicated success. It included a natural (although the correct word to be using is vaginal because inherent in the word "natural" is bias and judgment of whatever is deemed to not be "natural.") delivery with no medicine, effortless exclusive breastfeeding, and a quick discharge home.

I was checking none of the right boxes.

*   *   *

The days hospitalized and waiting for answers were just awful. The ward was overcrowded and overheated. It was June and it was unusually hot for England. The windows did not open because of sterilization and there was no air conditioning.

I felt like I was being suffocated.

The days are blurred in my memory so I don't remember the exact moment, but I remember the feeling when Giles told me that I wasn't going to be able to eat my placenta after all. There was too much meconium so it was tainted.

My placenta was tainted.

I was tainted.

I was unspooling by the hour but I didn't know it. Perhaps I was too numb, too tired, too shocked. Perhaps it was all of the above.

Giles was in and out, checking on the puppy at home and stopping to pick up fresh fruits and healthy snacks from Whole Foods because he knew that was what I liked to eat.

One afternoon, I hit a breaking point. I found myself screaming from my hospital bed, "Help me! Help me! Please! Help me!" while jamming the call button on the remote attached to my bed. I was sobbing—about what? I don't know. I was probably incoherent.

"Something's wrong. Something's wrong with me! Help me!" I kept saying to the nurse that came in. "I need the doctor, can you get the doctor?"

I don't think I could explain with any detail what was wrong with me. I just felt—off. Overwhelmed. Terrified.

Panicked.

I was trapped in my bed, with multiple IVs connecting me to I don't even know what. I was not able to move freely.

My body was *revolting*.

My body *was* revolting.

By the time Giles returned, holding a bag of groceries, I had stopped shrieking but I was still sobbing. I saw someone—a nurse? A doctor?—pull him aside for a chat. What were they talking about?

Giles came to my bedside and I was ready to hear how worried he was about me, ready to give into my hysteria again.

"What happened?" he asked.

"I don't know. Something's wrong. I don't know if it's another infection or something wrong with my chest but I can't breathe and I feel—"

He quietly interrupted me, "You can't do that."

My sobs abruptly stopped as I heard the serious tenor of his voice. I searched his face.

"They know about your mom. About her mental illness. They asked me if you had mental health problems."

I didn't understand.

"It's in your file. You must have told them about her."

"Well, yes, they ask about your family history and that's one of the questions . . . why, what . . . why did they bring that up?"

"They think you might be unstable. You need to pull it together. Don't you want to get out of here? Soon?"

I nodded.

"Then you need to try. Try to stay calm. Nothing is wrong with you. It's all just a lot, I know it is. Let's just get through this and get home."

*   *   *

I'm still not totally certain what happened. It could have been as simple as my milk coming in. Nobody had told me that when your milk first comes in, you can get fever and chills or that it can frankly be painful! Your breasts can become engorged with milk which, for a first-time mother, is understandably at the very least strange, isn't it? I had only really seen breastfeeding portrayed as being lovely and bonding— the most natural thing. Hollywood actresses were even featured in magazine photoshoots wearing couture while breastfeeding!

It could have been a panic attack. At that point in my life, I had had two very distinct and very memorable panic attacks. The first had happened during my last semester at college, not yet having a job secured for after graduation and the second had happened when I was living in Hong Kong, in a volatile relationship. In both situations, I felt like my sense of reality was collapsing in on itself and I needed to get outside and run, run for my life.

That was one thing I was literally unable to do while lying in the hospital bed after giving birth—run. I was in pain. I could hardly walk. I was literally attached to the bed.

There was no escape.

*   *   *

It felt like I was living in a nightmare. I could never have expected the beginnings of motherhood to be like this. And it wasn't just me that was having a difficult experience.

One night, there was a mother walking through the ward shouting, "I want my baby back! Bring my baby back!"

I have no idea what happened that she wasn't with her baby in that moment, but I felt her rage and her terror. My guess is that her baby was in the NICU and she just wanted to see her baby, but maybe she wasn't allowed because it wasn't visiting hours. Did they have visiting limitations for mothers? I was also afraid that they had maybe taken her baby away from her *because* she was unstable. She sure seemed unstable, screaming through the ward like that, but what mother wouldn't be, if she had her baby taken away?

The NICU itself was devastating to behold. While it was incredible that these tiny, vulnerable little humans were being cared for and kept alive, it was incredibly difficult and shocking to see the state of these babies fighting to survive. It was heartbreaking to see their parents, helpless, hoping. There was one baby girl I will never forget. She weighed just 930 grams. She was in a closed incubator and her parents would be there, just watching her through the plastic, unable to hold her, unable to heal her.

Our baby kept needing heel pricks. A four-pronged shot to be able to test his blood. His heel was so tiny, and the midwife would have to squeeze out droplets of blood while he screamed.

I resented the NICU. Why did some babies have to end up there while other babies got to go home, totally fine and totally healthy? It wasn't fair. I knew I should be grateful that all of the NICU babies were being cared for and kept alive. I knew I should be grateful for medicine and all the health-care workers.

But I still hated all of it.

*   *   *

I spoke with NICU Nurse Sarah Chung, RN, BSN, HN-BC, and she said something so simple and so true: "I'll never forget what the educator said to my class that I was going through NICU training with. She said that every mom can have a 'birth plan.' The birth plan never goes as they want it to. And obviously the last place they want their baby is in the NICU."

Of course. I couldn't possibly be alone in feeling terrified and heartbroken that my baby was in the NICU. No mother would have had NICU anywhere in their birth plan. So why is there no infrastructure of mental health support for mothers—and fathers—going through such a devastating and scary experience?

Nurse Chung echoed these sentiments: "I think that every parent in the NICU should have some sort of counseling. I'm the holistic nurse for the unit, and a lot of the nurses feel like these parents need a support group or some trained professional to talk with them because I think the experience is traumatic. I keep mentioning it to the hospital admin and they think that the social worker is enough, but all of the social workers are also overwhelmed. It's the social worker that is with all the parents and the babies being born. Do you know how many moms are giving birth? The social workers can't follow up with all of them all the time."

NICU parents are literally moving through a crisis at a time of life they expected would be mostly joyful albeit amid hard work. New parents are told about the upcoming sleepless nights and never-ending loads of laundry, but ventilators, IVs, heartrate monitors? There needs to be a network of mental and emotional care for all that a NICU parent is navigating.

*   *   *

On our second to last day, though we didn't yet know when we would finally be discharged from the hospital, my husband proposed a plan for me to get some fresh air.

We asked to speak to the head midwife and we asked if it would be okay for me to walk out to the coffee shop in the hospital lobby. She looked at us with confusion.

"Of course it is," she said. "Why are you asking me?"

We were stunned.

"We had been told Leah can't leave the ward," my husband explained.

"I don't know who told you that, but you may most definitely leave. In fact, we encourage you to get walking. It will help with the healing of your scar."

"But, I haven't left the ward for 10 days! I was told I couldn't!"

"Your *baby* cannot leave the ward, but you certainly can. You just need to stay on hospital grounds. You can go outside; we just need you to be close in case the baby needs you."

I was both irritated and elated. Finally, a taste of freedom!

With each step away from the ward, I started feeling a little bit better, a little bit more *normal*. We took the elevator to the ground level and I started heading toward the coffee shop when I felt my husband pull my hand toward the hospital exit. I hesitated.

"What if they need me to come back?"

"Come on, we're not going to go far. They can handle him for a bit. They know what they're doing more than we do!"

I was nervous, but also desperate to get outside. I looked at my husband and said, "Okay, let's do it."

We went through the sliding doors and into the parking lot. I assumed we would just take some slow laps around the hospital.

But Giles pulled me a different way.

"Wait! Where are we going?"

"Come on! There's a pub right up there. It's not far, I promise."

"A pub?! I can't go to a pub!"

"Why not? Let's have some food, and maybe even a cheeky drink?"

It did sound good. I looked up and noticed the windows of the NICU. I knew our baby was in safe hands.

"Okay, okay, but let's be quick!"

*   *   *

It felt like I had stepped into a different realm. The world had just been carrying on as normal this whole time? I couldn't process it. My entire everything had changed but nothing outside of me seemed to have changed. How did I fit into reality anymore?

All birth is traumatic, even without birth trauma in the sense of the baby's or mother's lives having been in danger. The National Institute of Mental Health (NIMH) defines a traumatic event as "a shocking, scary, or dangerous experience that can affect someone emotionally or physically."[3] We tend to only consider events that we would categorize as "bad" as being traumatic, and having a child is almost always framed as a blessing to be celebrated. And while it is indeed a blessing, most new parents will also feel overwhelmed, worried, confused, uncertain, and oh-so-tired.

According to the NIMH, experiencing these feelings in the first two weeks is considered "baby blues" whereas anything beyond that time period possibly indicates postpartum depression: "'Baby blues' is a term used to describe mild and short-lasting mood changes and feelings of worry, unhappiness, and exhaustion that many women experience in the first two weeks after giving birth. Babies require around-the-clock care, so it's normal for new mothers to feel tired or overwhelmed sometimes. Mood changes and feelings of anxiety or unhappiness that are severe or last longer than two weeks after childbirth may be signs of postpartum depression. Women with postpartum depression generally will not feel better without treatment."[4]

I don't know a single mother who only experienced mood changes, worry, and exhaustion for just the two-week period after childbirth. I know it doesn't mean that every single mother ends up with severe and debilitating depression, but it feels reasonable to think the challenge is considerable for most of us and that an infrastructure of maternal mental health support for all mothers is essential.

It is also a shock to go from the in-depth sometimes almost excessive prenatal care we receive to literally no postpartum care for the mother. Aside from one six-week checkup I had to confirm that my cesarian scar was not infected, all of the medical visits were now just for the baby.

The six-week checkup was also only part of the process of healing after the surgery. According to the NHS guidelines, "A Caesarean section is a major operation. It will take some time for you to return to normal. The outside skin edges of your wound should seal after about two days but the internal healing of muscle and other tissue below the surface goes on for many months."[5]

Many months. I wasn't facing just potentially two weeks of baby blues or six weeks of healing after cesarian. Many months.

Nobody told me that it would be many months. It makes me think that society just needs the mother to feel better as quickly as possible, despite her own physical and mental well-being, to just push through for the sake of the baby, the family unit, the status quo. And while this may lead to some semblance of success and survival in the short term, there is undoubtedly a cost in the long term, borne not just by the mother, but by her children and her partner as well.

*   *   *

When we were finally discharged and after we had packed up our belongings and secured the baby into his car seat in preparation to take him outside of the hospital for the first time since that sunny day eleven days prior, my husband and I looked at each other as if to say, "Now what?"

Were they really going to let us leave with this vulnerable human being? Were they really entrusting us with keeping him safe and alive? Was there at least a handbook they were going to send us home with?

A midwife walked by and I called out, "Excuse me? So, we can just go?"

With a knowing look, she said, "Of course!"

"Like, we can just leave, with the baby?"

"Of course you can! It's your baby!"

It felt completely irrational. We had no idea what we were doing! In no other role in life are you just thrown into it with such full responsibility and no training, and the stakes have never been higher. If that doesn't feel shocking and scary, I don't know what is.

For the mother in particular, there is the added layer of having experienced the physical and physiological changes that come with pregnancy and giving birth as well as the aftermath—the literal and metaphorical afterbirth. I minimized my concerns about it all by telling myself that billions of women have experienced this throughout all of human history . . . how hard could it be?

Nowadays, when I see a TV show where a new baby has been born into the family, I see how dishonest and incomplete the portrayal of this season of life typically is. The baby hardly cries, the parents' lives seem to carry on not too differently from before, and the mother inevitably, and effortlessly, always bounces back. Sometimes the baby is just never in the scene and I find myself shouting at the TV, "Who is with the baby right now?" Because if the parents are not, then some coordination of caretakers has had to have happened and who are the caretakers? Grandparents? Nannies? Babysitters? If a family relies on paid help, how much does it cost, and what is the story of financial privilege that enables the family to hire help?

When you add onto this reality a birth that required any combination of unwanted intervention, the need for the NICU, difficulty breastfeeding, a painful healing process, among many other things that can feel traumatic, it is no wonder that we are in a maternal mental health crisis.

2

Alien

Filling out intake forms at my first-ever prenatal appointment, I found myself stuck, unable to accurately identify myself. My options were: Caucasian. Afro-Caribbean. Chinese. Malaysian. Indian. Singaporean.

"Excuse me," I said to the midwife. "I don't have a box I can check."

She glanced at the paper I was holding and then glanced at my face, as if to fit my features into one of the choices on offer.

"You're not Chinese?"

"No, I'm Korean."

"Korean . . . that's not on here."

"Yes, that's what I'm saying."

"Can you check Singaporean?"

"But I'm not Singaporean, I'm Korean."

"Well, just pick one, it doesn't really matter."

When I tell people here in the United States that I had my first child in the United Kingdom, there are assumptions that everything must have been great because the United Kingdom has socialized healthcare—the NHS. America, of course, is well known for its health-care-for-profit system. But from my very first prenatal appointment, I understood that the system—even one that was available for everyone—was not really designed for people that look like me.

When I tell my friends in the United States that I was sent home from the hospital even after it was confirmed that all my waters were gone, most of them are shocked. The standard here is that you would be admitted immediately, because the baby should be born within twenty-four hours. They would want to monitor both you and the baby. The medical perspective is that without the protection of the amniotic sac, the baby is at risk of infection, a risk that proceeds to grow exponentially with each passing hour.

There is criticism that our modern society is overly medical and medicated. I personally do believe in the inherent wisdom of our bodies. So I did not think to question it when they sent me home—I figured my body would just do what was necessary.

I also assumed that it was just done differently in the United Kingdom, that it was just less medicalized than the United States, which felt like a good thing. But a month after my son was born, a friend of mine in London had a similar experience with her water breaking before having any contractions. Because she knew what I had been through, and also probably because this was her second baby, when she went to the hospital, she refused to leave. She wanted to make sure the baby would be delivered within twenty-four hours. She advocated for herself and she was accepted and admitted. She had a straightforward vaginal delivery with no complications. Both she and her baby were perfectly healthy.

She—and her baby—are white.

*   *   *

The story of my own birth has been told and retold in our family. I was supposed to be named Leonardo (after Da Vinci—my father is an artist/inventor) because I was expected to be a boy. My dad had picked up *It's a Boy!* cigars and brought a baseball mitt to the hospital, awaiting the arrival of his firstborn son. In Korean culture, having a firstborn son is considered fortuitous—a guarantee of the continuation of the family name.

Everyone was shocked to see that I was, in fact, a girl.

I always wondered how it could have been possible that they didn't know I was a girl and not a boy. I was born in 1980—ultrasound had already been invented and regularly used to monitor pregnancies.

"I don't know," my mom would say. "They just saw it wrong, I guess."

I think, now, that there must have been a lot lost in translation. Although my parents have lived in the United States for nearly fifty years, they will always be Korean first. Their mother tongue will always be Korean.

As well, I can't help but wonder how they were viewed and treated by the medical staff overseeing my mother's pregnancy. Who were the doctors and nurses who saw her? Did they see a human being worthy of care? She has always spoken English with an accent and it would have been clear that she was not American. Were they careless? Was that why she, too, ended up getting an emergency cesarian?

And what mental health support could there have been for an immigrant like my mother? Did she ever really understand why she needed the emergency surgery? Did she feel seen within the system at all? What did her community look like once she took her new baby home, figuring out how to be a mother in a country that was not her own, that did not value her as they do white mothers?

I will never know for sure when her depression started, but after having gone through my own postpartum depression, I think it's likely that hers started during this postpartum period as well. And as much as we see today that there is no systemic infrastructure of maternal mental health care, we can know that it would have been that much more nonexistent decades ago.

*		*		*

For years, I ruminated on the birth of my son. I played out different scenarios, wishing for the impossible—for things to have turned out differently. I shamed myself for not being able to snap out of it. The baby and I were healthy now—wasn't that all that mattered?

Once, a friend said to me: "Are you really that bothered that you needed a cesarian? I don't think I would have cared."

I felt so hurt by this. It seemed a rather insensitive comment coming from someone who herself had fulfilled her birth plan of a water birth.

According to the National Childbirth Trust, the UK's national charity for pregnancy, birth, and early parenthood, "Many people feel unprepared for their birth experience and as many as one in three people report feeling traumatized after giving birth. . . . Feeling upset or distressed by what happened when you were giving birth may mean you're experiencing birth trauma. Every person's experience is different, but trauma can be triggered by both physical and emotional experiences. It might be that your birth was long and intense, that you had an unplanned intervention, that you weren't looked after or listened to in labor, or perhaps there were concerns about the safety of you or your baby."[1]

If one in three people experience birth trauma, why was I not having this conversation with health-care workers or even with friends? Why is there no infrastructure of support? Surely any birth that ends up in emergency surgery should at the very least come with an info sheet on how to spot possible signs of feeling traumatized, like the info sheets given if we opt for any vaccines?

Instead, you're gaslight with platitudes:

At least you have a healthy baby.

At least you're healthy.

At least you *have* a baby.

At least you didn't die.

Trauma is not what happens to you, but what happens within you as a response to what you experience. But this is not colloquially understood, leading to conversations that may unintentionally cause harm, furthering the trauma. Your experience may be compared against another mother who may have had a very similar birth, but for a possible plethora of reasons, did not experience trauma.

The circumstances could have been exactly the same but for one factor. Maybe the baby did not have an infection and had to go to the NICU. Maybe that mother didn't have a job that relied on her body. Maybe she had the support of her own mother and her closest friends from childhood. Maybe her husband had a longer paternity leave.

Maybe, maybe, maybe.

Almost exactly five years after I had my first child, one of my longtime friends gave birth to her first. She, like me, had wanted a "natural" birth.

When she went into labor, her husband was keeping everyone, including me, up to date with text messages. Hours and eventually a night passed. Finally, I received a photo of their new baby with the news that everything was good and that my friend was recovering well from a cesarian. My heart sank. I was instantly worried about how she would be feeling. I assumed she would be feeling traumatized like I had.

But she wasn't traumatized.

She was disappointed, sure. But that was just a background feeling for her. Her main emotional state was of maternal jubilation. She felt instantly bonded to her daughter and this connection just grew over time. She co-slept, loved breastfeeding, and reveled in becoming a mother.

I was happy, if envious, for her. I was also completely perplexed. How could we have such different responses to needing an unplanned cesarian birth? I internalized it as a failure on my part. Maybe I wasn't grateful enough. Maybe I was too controlling. What was wrong with me?

In one of our many conversations about all things motherhood, my friend said something that helped alchemize my trauma. She told me that she thinks it is precisely because she knew what I had been through that she was able to process her experience better. Needing a cesarian despite really hoping for a vaginal delivery was something she was aware could happen. She also knew that it didn't mean failure, or that her bond with her child would be any less, or that it said anything about her potential as a mother. Because she saw in me a mother who cared deeply about her child, irrespective of the way the child had been born. This enduring motherly love was what was important, not what happened on the day the baby arrived.

I also can't help but wonder how our racial identities could have played into how we felt we were being treated, not just at the birth but throughout our maternal care. My friend and her child are white. As a person of color, you are never not aware that you are not white. We all figure out how we can survive in this system that places whiteness above all other identities, this system of white supremacy. How can we assimilate? How can we become as white adjacent as possible? How can we safeguard our humanity?

As a second-generation Asian American who grew up middle class, I know I am not the most oppressed in the context of systemic racism. I am aware that whiteness gives me more permission to exist than it does to my Black, brown, and Indigenous siblings. And that is precisely why I feel it is my duty to speak about the systemic injustices that persist, especially when it comes to fellow mothers and our children.

Dr. Uché Blackstock writes about her experience as a pregnant Black woman in her book *Legacy: A Black Physician Reckons with Racism in Medicine*. Her happiness about expecting her first baby lived alongside her anxiety about how she knew the system saw her.

"Throughout my medical education, differences between Black and white patients were passed off as information, as data, as the objective truth. No one made the point that using race as an aid in diagnosis might lead to bias and stereotyping, which in turn could lead to misdiagnosis, thereby harming Black patients . . . the reality is that racism absolutely exists in medicine, it's existed throughout history, and it's still hurting—and often killing—Black Americans."[2]

Dr. Blackstock was well aware that despite her privileges and being a doctor herself, the odds were unjustly against her simply based on her racial identity. She knew she was "still five times more likely to die in childbirth than a white birthing person with the same qualifications" because "the hard truth is that inequitable maternal health outcomes for Black birthing people persist across socioeconomic backgrounds and educational levels."[3]

She continues, "The statistics are staggering. To this day, the United States spends more on health care and births than any other country in the world, but it also has one of the highest maternal mortality rates of any high-income nation. These numbers are in large part driven by the high Black maternal mortality rate, with Black birthing people three to four times more likely to die of pregnancy-related complications than white birthing people. In NYC . . . the Black maternal mortality rate is nine times as high as it is for their white peers."[4]

Nine times as high.

Dr. Blackstock goes on to offer the following comparisons:

Black birthing people, when compared to white counterparts, in the United States are twice as likely to:

- have a preterm birth;

- give birth to a low-birth-weight baby;

- have a child that dies before the age of one;

- be ignored by a health-care professional when they report symptoms or ask for help.

Furthermore:

- Twenty-two percent of Black birthing people report being mistreated by a health-care professional during pregnancy and childbirth.

- Black birthing people are 36 percent more likely to have a C-section than birthing people of other races, which increases the risk of mortality.

- Preeclampsia is 60 percent more common, and it is a leading cause of mortality.

- Black birthing people across socioeconomic status are least likely to nurse compared to all races, and we must consider "the deep trauma of slavery, in which enslaved women were forced to wet-nurse their enslavers' babies."[5]

These statistics are deeply alarming and indicate that we are far from a racially equal society, even when it comes to the basic human right of health care during one of the most important times of a person's life—bringing a child into the world. Our society claims to prioritize care of the most vulnerable people. On public transportation, there are special seats for people with young children, people who are pregnant, and the elderly. And yet, the numbers tell a different story, one that cannot be separated from a racialized reality.

New York-based NICU nurse Sarah Chung corroborates these statistics based on her experience on the ground: "I think in terms of race and/or ethnicity, a lot of the patients that we deal with only speak Spanish. And I feel like they are treated differently. If they are not Spanish speaking, they are Black and/or they speak Bengali or Arabic, languages that are less likely to be represented by our staff, even as diverse as our nursing staff is. And I do feel like these patients are treated differently if only because it's harder with a language barrier. It shouldn't impede on the care, but it does sometimes."

Nurse Chung agreed that it was accurate to say that the NICU had a disproportionately higher number of families of color than white families. I wanted to understand better why this is the case.

She explained, "I think that's a separate discussion on economics, because a lot of our NICU patients have comorbidities like high blood pressure, kidney disease, sickle cell disease . . . all these other health conditions that definitely affect a mother during her pregnancy. Based on what we see in our NICU, it would seem that white mothers have more access to healthier food and more money to take care of themselves."

It is heartbreaking and enraging to realize that systemic racism—which impacts a family's socioeconomic status—leads to medical injustices that can negatively impact the health of innocent babies. Pregnant women of color face less care and more stress at multiple stages of pregnancy. How can we trust the medical system to keep us safe?

I don't know that mothers of color can safely rely on the system as it is now. I think we have to build our own communities of care. We have to take our experiences and skills and what we understand about how these systems are failing us and build new spaces where marginalized identities are centered and protected.

Psychotherapist and NICU mom Melissa Bada-Devers, LCSW, has dedicated her holistic therapy practice to empowering people of color because of what she has experienced and witnessed as a person of color and as the daughter of immigrants: "My clients who are Black mothers—including someone who herself is a doula—are very traumatized about going to a hospital. They are very traumatized about going to give birth. They are very traumatized even without their own experiences because they know how they will be treated. Growing up, I saw how my own mom was treated when we went to the ER, and the only reason that they changed their attitude with her was because my mom was an RN. Otherwise if you're Hispanic and if you're still speaking Spanish, you automatically get judged more. This is why now my whole clientele is clients of color. They are sons and daughters of immigrants."

I believe we have to take care of each other. We have to weave a tapestry of collective care outside of the systems, that can scaffold and safeguard us where systems fail us. Collective includes everyone— of all identities. But the most marginalized identities must be centered and uplifted, because once we reach a point where our most marginalized are truly cared for, we will know that we have built the capacity to care for all of us. And I believe the wellness of any society has to be rooted in the protection of the children, and therefore the health—physical and otherwise—of the caregivers.

*   *   *

My daughter, our second child, was born near the end of 2020 when we were deep in social distancing. For our baby gift, my father offered to pay for us to hire a baby nurse for a few weeks. Our son was still doing remote learning, and I think most parents that experienced this period know how challenging it was to keep your kids engaged, let alone actually learning, in Zoom school. Especially with my history of postpartum depression, I was terrified to attempt to go through the newborn season without any help, so I was grateful for my father's generous gift.

Our baby nurse, Pearl, is just a gem of a human being. She is from Trinidad, radiates the most motherly warmth, and tells the best stories. We loved her immediately. She took Covid as seriously as we did, and although it was different from how she normally worked as a baby nurse, we decided that she would move in for the few weeks that she was with us, to minimize potential exposure risk outside of our bubble. And so when the Covid vaccine first became available for her age group, I was surprised that she told us that she was not going to get it.

I had never questioned any vaccine that a doctor had prescribed, whether for myself or for my children. I was aware of the anti-vax movement, but it always felt conspiratorial to me. Pearl had seemed so practical and wise and I knew she took her health and the health of the babies she took care of very seriously. I wondered and asked, what was going on?

She explained, "I am very weary of the American healthcare system. I just don't trust what they are saying."

"But this is just science, isn't it?" I asked.

"Science for whose benefit? You know what they did at Tuskegee. I don't trust the medical system."

Tuskegee? It sounded ever so vaguely familiar, but really, I had no idea what she was talking about. And of course I didn't—it was by design that I didn't. Much of our racist history is left out of history books and continues to be censored today, as we see in book bans and an increasing divestment from DEI initiatives across all sectors.

In a McGill Office for Science and Society article called "40 Years of Human Experimentation in America: The Tuskegee Study," Ada McVean writes, "The 'Tuskegee Study of Untreated Syphilis in the Negro Male,' was conducted by the United States Public Health Service. . . . The goal was to 'observe the natural history of untreated syphilis' in [B]lack populations. But the subjects were unaware of this and were simply told they were receiving treatment for bad blood. Actually, they received no treatment at all. Even after penicillin was discovered as a safe and reliable cure for syphilis, the majority of men did not receive it."[6]

Further in the article, McVean offers the societal context of racism: "Before the ending of slavery, scientific racism was used to justify the African slave trade. Scientists argue that African men were uniquely fit for enslavement due to their physical strength and simple minds. They argued that slaves possessed primitive nervous systems, so did not experience pain as white people did. Enslaved African Americans in the South were claimed to suffer from mental illness at rates lower than their free Northern counterparts . . . and slaves who ran away were said to be suffering from their own mental illness known as drapetomania."[7]

Drapetomania was a proposed new disease that Dr. Samuel Cartwright attempted to create in 1851. The medical journal The Lancet defines drapetomania as a discarded diagnosis that "was derived from two Greek words, one meaning 'a runaway slave', the other signifying 'mad or crazy'. This mental disorder of slaves had one defining characteristic: the sufferer had an unconscionable desire to abscond from his or her owner."[8]

The attempt to categorize a person's desire for freedom and for their humanity to be respected as a mental illness is as absurd as it is racist. That a physician could even attempt to create a disease based on such nonsense speaks to the level of dehumanization that Black folks in our country have always had to fight against.

Returning to McVean's article, we can understand even more about the history of the official American perception of Black people: "Scientific and medical authorities of the late 19th/ early 20th centuries held extremely harmful pseudoscientific ideas specifically about the sex drives and genitals of African Americans. It was widely believed that, while the brains of African Americans were under-evolved, their genitals were over-developed. Black men were seen to have an intrinsic perversion for white women, and all African Americans were seen as inherently immoral, with insatiable sexual appetites. This all matters because it was with these understandings of race, sexuality and health that researchers undertook the Tuskegee study. They believed, largely due to their fundamentally flawed scientific understandings of race, that [B]lack people were extremely prone to sexually transmitted infections (like syphilis). Low birth rates and high miscarriage rates were universally blamed on STIs."[9]

Pearl had a rightful mistrust of science and our health-care system. How could she know for sure that any vaccine she agreed to get was indeed what it was claimed to be? Maybe it would be for certain people and maybe other people's bodies would be used as a testing ground.

How many other medical crimes such as the Tuskegee so-called Study have happened that just never broke through to the mainstream? How many are still continuing to this day?

And what is the impact on a person's mental health to know that people who look like them are quite literally considered to be expendable?

Even fame and wealth do not insulate people of color. Consider Serena Williams' birth story. In the April 2022 issue of Elle Magazine, Williams writes about her experience having to advocate for herself immediately after the birth of her first child: "I couldn't breathe. I was coughing because I just couldn't get enough air. . . . I was coughing because I had an embolism, a clot in one of my arteries. The doctors would also discover a hematoma, a collection of blood outside the blood vessels, in my abdomen, then even more clots that had to be kept from traveling to my lungs."[10]

Williams had insisted that she needed to have a CAT scan but was continually told that she just needed to rest. It was only when her nurse finally called her doctor who ordered a CAT scan that they were able to confirm that Williams had been right: "I had a blood clot in my lungs, and they needed to insert a filter into my veins to break up the clot before it reached my heart."[11]

Williams is a globally known and decorated athlete, a tennis champion with twenty-three Grand Slams to her name. It was only after multiple requests for further investigation into why she was coughing that she got the lifesaving treatment that she needed. But what if she hadn't finally received a "yes" amid all the invalidation?

Citing the statistics also mentioned by Dr. Blackstock that Black women are three times as likely to die during or after childbirth than their white counterparts, Williams writes: "Many of these deaths are considered by experts to be preventable. Being heard and appropriately treated was the difference between life or death for me; I know those statistics would be different if the medical establishment listened to every Black woman's experience."[12]

There are so many dangers to jumping to the assumption that we are living in a post-racial society where people claim to not see color. With the current administration's amplified attacks on immigrants and DEI, I wonder if and hope that a positive outcome might be that more of us see the truth, and that those of us who believe in the equality of all human beings irrespective of identity will more boldly speak up against injustice.

We cannot fix a problem that we are not aware of or that we won't admit exists. The accounts I have so far provided pertain specifically to the stories of Black birthing women because they are the ones most harmed within the medical system. I also believe that racism against any group is racism against every group—we are all in the same fight for equality, and I believe it is the responsibility of those that are afforded more privilege to stand up for those that are more at risk and silenced.

As a yoga practitioner of nearly thirty years, I understand that there is no separation between the body and the mind. I used to think that this meant I could mind control my body to do whatever I wanted. *If I think it, I will manifest it!* But I now understand that no, that is just the ego wanting to control everything.

The mind-body connection is about the deep relationship that exists between our mind—our thoughts, ideas, dreams, calculations, intellect—and our body—our skin, limbs, organs, gut, intuition. It is about the interconnectedness of our mental and physical health and well-being. Our mind and body are interdependent; they influence and impact each other constantly.

Williams listened to her body, intuited that something was wrong, and was listened to, eventually, when she advocated for herself.

Pearl made a decision that could influence her physical health because she knew from understanding this country's racist history that she could not trust what she was being told.

Dr. Blackstock knew from her medical studies, professional experience, and lived reality that she was not safe as a pregnant Black woman, and this caused her anxiety. In her book, she shares, "I thought a lot about weathering during my pregnancy, how internalizing the external stress of everyday racism manifests itself in our bodies."[13]

Stress manifests itself in our bodies.

There is no separation between the mind and the body.

When we are pregnant through to the fourth trimester period just after birth, we are at the behest of our medical care. What happens when we are not seen as fully human by the health-care professionals taking care of us? What happens when we are not listened to and believed? Even if there isn't a severe illness or crisis, the impact on our self-worth and sanity can be detrimental and long-lasting.

All during one of the most vulnerable and sleep-deprived periods of a mother's life. Yet we are expected to bounce back, to be happy, to spin all the plates. And this applies to all of us mothers irrespective of race.

When doula, writer, and mother Ashley Simpo was pregnant, she decided to switch out of the medical system and into the full-time care of a midwife. She had noticed an absence of questions from the doctors and nurses she saw in her early prenatal appointments that would have indicated that she was being seen as a whole human being. As a Black woman, she questioned what this meant about the care she would get: "I was never asked, do you feel any stress right now, or what are you feeling emotionally? Do you feel safe? Did you feel safe getting here? Anything that can make a doctor's visit more personal to that individual. I don't think that we're asking pregnant Black women the softer questions. I think it's more data driven questions. Like, are you in an abusive relationship? Let's look at your urine sample. And while those things are important to know about the physical health and vitality of the woman's body, your mind state and your emotional state have a huge effect on how your pregnancy is going to go, how you're managing stress, how you're sleeping. I had a couple doctor's visits when I was first pregnant and those visits were maybe 15 minutes each. When I saw my midwife, we were talking for 45 minutes. It was a conversation. I credit having, and I am really thankful that I had, an uncomplicated birth to the work that went into my mental and emotional state, rather than focusing just on what numbers are showing up on a chart."

How might the outcome of births be affected if the care we receive as pregnant women and people was more holistic, in the sense that we are not just a physical vessel but a whole universe, growing another whole universe within ourselves? What if we felt more seen for all the layers of our humanity? What if we connected the dots of racism, white supremacy, individualism, and other systems of oppression to what literally manifests in our own lives, minds, and bodies?

I think that is where we find our liberation.

Simpo knew she could not take for granted that she would be cared for by the medical system: "I had learned about the history of births in hospitals and generally how Black women have been treated, such as with the use of Norplant and requiring Black women on welfare to be on Norplant in order to have support and the history of trying to control Black women's ability to give birth. I learned that the history of gynecology wouldn't exist without Black enslaved women—we wouldn't have the speculum. The origin of gynecology is steeped in the production of slaves. They discovered a lot of gynecological advancements through experimenting on Black women's bodies without consent or with coercion. It's steeped in a really dark and ugly history. And that means when I walk into the gynecologist's office, I know why it exists. I know what I need from it and what I don't need from it. I know I should do my own research before I get there. I know that a gynecologist is maybe my last resort after I've talked to a midwife or an herbalist or my aunt.

"It's really important for anyone with a womb to understand that these systems are steeped in a really oppressive history. We need to make sure we know what we're doing here and if we should be here and what we need, and make sure to walk out with what we need. I think that's one of the reasons why you do need an advocate in the room."

Indeed, as Simpo says, the history of gynecology is oppressive and deeply disturbing. Gynecology was fathered by Dr. James Marion Sims. Dr. Sims experimented on Black female slaves who had no rights, including the right to consent. What's important to recognize is that what happened in history—a history that was not that long ago in the mid-1800s—continues to manifest in unequal care for Black Americans today. As reported on NPR, "Black patients continue to receive less pain medication for broken bones and cancer.

Black children receive less pain medication than white children for appendicitis. One reason for this is that many people inaccurately believe that [B]lacks literally have thicker skin than whites and experience less pain."[14]

The enduring dehumanization of Black bodies is unacceptable and we as conscientious members of the collective must vehemently reject anything that puts our kin—of any and all identities—at unjust and unnecessary risk. We need to keep educating ourselves and learning the history of how we got here.

Dr. Vanessa Northington Gamble is a physician and medical historian at George Washington University who teaches a course on the history of race and racism in American medicine. Dr. Gamble was interviewed for the NPR Hidden Brain podcast episode that was published on February 7, 2017. She says, "Starting in 1845, [Sims] started to conduct experiments on enslaved women. And why we talk about Sims today . . . is that he perfected a technique to repair a condition called vesicovaginal fistula . . . [which] basically means that there is an opening between the vagina and also the bladder or the vagina and the rectum, which usually comes after traumatic childbirth. And Sims started a series of experiments to repair these fistulas.

"These women were property. These women could not consent. These women also had value to the slaveholders for production and reproduction—how much work they could do in the field, how many enslaved children they could produce. And by having these fistulas, they could not continue with childbirth and also have difficulty working.

"[The surgeries] were performed without anesthesia. There was a belief at the time that [B]lack people did not feel pain in the same way. They were not vulnerable to pain, especially [B]lack women. [T]his surgery was done where [B]lack women were naked. So when we think about it, I think we think about pain. We also need to think about how these women's dignity was also taken away from them.

"He did treat white women. But he treated white women with anesthesia. . . . But the technique had been perfected on the bodies of [B]lack women."[15]

I think about what I learned through Dr. Blackstock's book *Legacy*, Serena Williams' birth story, and the Tuskegee Study. Medicine— including and especially obstetrics and gynecology—continues to be a racist institution. Where does that leave us mothers of color?

I had not known any of this history of gynecology in this country. I had not known about the controversy with Norplant that Simpo mentioned, which was FDA approved in 1990 and discontinued in 2002. All of this is very recent history.

In an essay titled *The Norplant Solution: Norplant and the Control of African-American Motherhood*, peer-reviewed and published in the *UCLA WOMEN'S LAW JOURNAL* in 1995, Darci Elaine Burrell wrote: "The individuals behind the Norplant 'bonus' programs see the regulation of poor, African-American women's reproductive freedom as a solution to social problems, primarily the 'welfare mess.' The 'welfare mess' consists of African-American welfare mothers, generational welfare dependency, and the violent, mostly Black inner city.

"Across the country, legislatures also see the 'induced' use of Norplant as a solution to the 'welfare mess.' All fifty states have included the contraceptive in their Medicaid programs to some degree. All states and the District of Columbia now reimburse poor women for the cost of Norplant, and some states have proposed offering cash incentives for the use of Norplant. The Governor of Maryland has even suggested that Norplant should be mandatory for women on welfare. Under a plan proposed in Kansas, AFDC recipients would receive a free Norplant implant along with a $500 cash grant. Recipients would also be entitled to a $50 grant for every year they kept the implant."[16]

While it can be tempting to compartmentalize the history of slavery, eugenics, and forced sterilization as having been from a different time, it is impossible to ignore what has been happening in our own lifetime. The National Black Women's Reproductive Justice Agenda reported on the blatant racism of the use of Norplant to control and limit the fertility of Black women as well as other marginalized communities including women of color, immigrant women, and women with low incomes or disabilities. "Family planning decisions were often made *for* Black women, not *by* Black women, with the goal of either controlling Black women and their reproduction or advancing contraceptive research at Black women's expense."[17]

Simpo was right. It is imperative to know our history. It may not always be readily available—in fact, sometimes it's designed to be hidden from us. But as ever, knowledge is our empowerment and as women—and especially as mothers—we need to be empowered for one another, for our collective motherhood.

Simpo was moved to become a protective presence and advocate for other mothers and ultimately became certified as a doula: "I think what really launched my decision was when Roe v Wade was overturned and I was the managing editor at *CRWNMAG* at the time. I was interviewing a full spectrum doula and two seconds into the call is when we found out about Roe v Wade being overturned. Our whole conversation shifted. Everything felt devastating. What they said is what made me want to become a doula. They said, 'Nobody can take away something that wasn't theirs to take.'

"We have always inherently known how to care for our village, for our people, for our bodies, from way before there was a Roe v Wade. And so it is going to be about education and getting back to a kind of indigenous grass roots understanding and knowledge of our body.

We are going to have to really learn a lot about ourselves in order to sustain our communities and each other as we watch these systems that we have known fall away and break apart.

"It made me realize how important it is for there to be someone in the room who is reminding you that your body belongs to you and not to this doctor or to this hospital. And when you see a mother who does feel empowered about birth and about her experience, feelings and whatever it is she's experiencing versus someone who is just reliant on whatever they're being told and desperate and just wanting to get through it, it's like a light switches on. I realized that this is radical work."

The radical work of motherhood. This was precisely the alchemy I was searching for. In the same way that I have been connecting the dots of lived, generational, and systemic traumas, Simpo has been connecting the dots of history, the current political climate, and our bodies as women and mothers. We simply cannot separate ourselves from the systems that we live in so it's imperative that we understand what they are and how they impact us. We also need to bring one another into this work. This is how we build our power and how we safeguard our physical and mental well-being.

As much as I would like to believe otherwise, it is likely too much to think that our entire medical infrastructure can be reformed and many if not most of us don't have access to hiring our own midwives or doulas. But the more we as mothers and expectant mothers understand the ways in which we are often failed, the more we can advocate for ourselves and for each other. The more power we can take back in keeping each other safe.

For those mothers of color that survive all the statistics stacked against us, there lingers a mistrust, fear, and isolation. These feelings can't help but be transferred to your child, too, who likely looks more like you than like the white children that our country more easily values. The mental weight of not fully knowing if you can trust your health care professionals to care about the health and well-being of you and your child is immense. Most parents are often fully reliant on our pediatricians to properly diagnose symptoms and prescribe medications and recovery plans. We are at the mercy of our doctors.

Cycles of harm continue when they are not addressed, admitted, and accounted for. I actually believe in the good of most people. I don't believe we come into this world hating others. Hate and divisiveness are taught, both explicitly and implicitly. There is an undercurrent of rationalizations that get us to a point of seeing aliens rather than kin in someone that is of a different identity, and although I am focusing on race here, this applies to all marginalized identities when it comes to gender, sexual orientation, body size, disability, neurodivergence, and more.

I don't know if I will live to see the eradication of racism and white supremacy. These ideologies are multipronged and deeply rooted. The good fight has been ongoing, carried through history by many revolutionary souls.

What I do know is that I can keep pushing the conversation forward as a mother, starting with how I raise my own children.

I have always spoken to my children about how we are all different and how these differences are amazing and beautiful. I have made a concerted effort to build a life of diversity—a rainbow of humans. This is easier to do here in New York City than in many other places in this country. Just the regular exposure to a variety of ethnicities, foods, and languages is normalizing, and you tend to come to appreciate differences rather than fear them.

Culture has definitely shifted from when I was a child; I noticed a book at my daughter's preschool called *Sunday Funday in Koreatown*—and I was not the one to have brought it in! It's deeply heartwarming to know that there are others in our community with shared values.

We need to keep going. We need to keep driving culture. Multicultural books and other forms of media are a beautiful beginning to understanding and celebrating that we are all one human race, but we need to push beyond representation. Yes, it means something to me that Michelle Yeoh, an Asian American woman, won the Best Actress Oscar in 2023. Yes, I am touched when non-Koreans tell me about their favorite Korean foods, spas, and dramas.

And I want to know: What are you doing to understand the lived experience of those with different identities than you? How are you advocating for equal rights for all? Do you speak up when you witness racism and other forms of injustice? Do you talk to your loved ones about these uncomfortable truths?

We all need to be doing this work, whether or not we feel that we are from marginalized identities or that we are personally affected. As an Asian American, one of my responsibilities is to fight against anti-Blackness within my community. I believe such interracial division and competition have been laid on us by white supremacy, which manufactures scarcity—scarcity of resources and jobs but most of all, scarcity of white acceptance.

White supremacy has to reckon with us people of color because it is a fact that we exist, and that we exist in far greater numbers than whiteness. Author and educator Rosemary M. Campbell-Stephens coined the idea of the Global Majority, defining it as follows: "Global Majority is a collective term. It refers to people who identity as Black, African, Asian, Brown, Arab, mixed-heritage, are indigenous to the global south, and or, have been routinely racialised as 'ethnic-minorities'. Globally, these groups currently represent approximately eighty-five per cent (85%) of the world's population making them the global majority now, and with current growth rates notwithstanding Covid-19 and its emerging variants, the global majority is set to remain so for the foreseeable future."[18]

We people of color despite often being relegated to "minorities" are actually the majority in the global context. This means that we have more power than we think. And the more that we can focus on the fact that as different as we may feel from each other, we have one major commonality—the same oppressor—the stronger we will be. This means joining together in our struggles. We have to care about the rights of our fellow people of the global majority as much as we care about our own.

It is also important to note Campbell-Stephens' disclaimer that COVID-19 could potentially impact the growth rate of the global majority. Remembering Nurse Chung's observation that a mother's socioeconomic status impacts her ability to keep herself and her children healthy, we must consider who has been most at risk of dying of COVID-19.

As reported by the Mayo Clinic, "In the early years of the COVID-19 pandemic, American Indian and Alaska Native people, non-Hispanic Black people and Hispanic people had higher rates of infection and COVID-19 deaths compared with those of non-Hispanic white people. Black and Hispanic people in the United States also had higher chances of needing care in the hospital for COVID-19."[19]

Similarly, a University of College London report found clear racialized outcomes in England:

"The report found that ethnic minority and migrant communities faced:

- Increased vulnerability: Depending on the ethnic group, individuals were found to be between 5% and 88% more likely to contract the virus. This alarming disparity underscored the urgent need for targeted interventions to address the specific challenges faced by these communities, the report said.

- Excess deaths: By April 2022, the end of community testing, Asian communities in England had over 10,500 excess deaths and Black communities almost 6,000. These are people who would likely have been alive were it not for the pandemic. Black and Asian communities had around a 23% higher risk of experiencing excess deaths and the same trend exists for other ethnic groups too.

- Limited access to sick pay: Black, Asian, and minority ethnic workers were found to have less access to sick pay, while undocumented workers had no access to it at all. This lack of financial protection not only compromised the health and wellbeing of individuals but also perpetuated the spread of the virus within these communities.

- Inadequate support schemes: Many Black, Asian, and minority ethnic individuals reported limited support from existing schemes. This insufficiency exacerbated the economic and social hardships faced by these communities, hindering their ability to cope with the pandemic's impact effectively.

- Unequal vaccination coverage: The vaccination programme failed to reach migrants and Black, Asian, and minority ethnic communities adequately, leaving them without the same level of protection as their White British counterparts. This disparity threatened to prolong the pandemic and perpetuated health disparities among different demographic groups.

The report underscored the urgent need for evidence-based policies and practices that prioritise the needs of Black, ethnic minority and migrant communities. It called for a comprehensive and inclusive approach that addresses the systemic barriers to healthcare access, ensures equitable distribution of resources, and tackles the underlying social determinants of health."[20]

The glaring inequities in the impact of the pandemic can be traced right back to the roots of white supremacy. It is not an exaggeration to say that the less privilege you have in the system of whiteness, the more likely you are to have inadequate health care which can result in poor mental health, job loss, and death.

*   *   *

As I researched statistics for this chapter, I found that it was much easier to find information on Black maternal statistics than other racialized minorities. I believe this is part of the interracial division to keep us in our separate corners, not realizing we are actually all in the same fight.

Consider that the March of Dimes reports that the "maternal death rate for pregnant Black _and_ American Indian/Alaska Native people is about three times higher than it is for white people who are pregnant. These disparities increase by age. The maternal death rate of Black and American Indian/Alaska Native pregnant people who are 30 years old or older is about four to five times higher than it is for white people who are pregnant. This is not acceptable."[21]

Indeed, none of this is acceptable and the truth of such statistics materializes into mental health symptoms for mothers such as T'lingit Indigenous non-binary climate activist, artist, and educator Roberta Sam:

A lot of Native women have very high medical anxiety. We all know that disclosing that I am Native could get me killed or could get my children taken away. Birth alerts still happen in Canada.

I myself have very intense medical anxiety. I have a very big distrust when it comes to the system, because the more I learn of it, the more I understand how it was in many ways intentionally set up to exploit people like me—Alaskan and other marginalized populations too. Learning about my history, Alaska's history, I see how they criminalized mental health and mental illness.

I nearly died the first time I gave birth. I wish I had a better experience. My midwife appointments were great. In Washington State, we have midwives and nurses pretty much the whole time. All the women I interacted with were great. But when I gave birth the first time, I had an anxiety attack in the middle of labor. I started losing it and my heart rate was getting concerning. A doctor who hadn't so much as poked his head in the whole time, during the several hours I had been there at that point, suddenly announced, "All right this one's going to get a c-section" and I knew he was talking about me. I didn't even have time to react before my midwife who had actually been with me the whole time, stood up and went right to the doctor. I could hear her screaming, "Let us do our job, you are not taking this one!" I remember her saying, "you are not taking this one" and knowing what I know now of how many Native women don't come back from C-sections, I'm convinced she saved my life.

I was not successful in finding statistics on what Sam shared with me, and I can't help but think that it is because that information is intentionally buried. The North American continent became what it is today because of the genocide of our Indigenous people, a genocide that continues on, albeit in a slower, quieter way. From boarding schools to orphan trains to starlight tours, the horrific dehumanization of and violence against Native people has never ended.

*   *   *

What happens when we broaden the scope of the conversation to unite all racialized minorities in the context of white supremacy? The common denominator would become much more obvious which means our fight for justice and liberation can become that much more strategic.

Race is often presented in a binary way, quite literally in the language of Black versus white. There are historical reasons for this, to be sure, as it was Black Africans that were brought to this land against their will and enslaved. But this land was also stolen from the Indigenous people and immigrants, whose own countries have often suffered because of Western imperialism and who have played and continue to play a critical role in keeping this country running.

I believe we need to move away from the idea of oppression Olympics. In fact, I believe that that framing is a decoy thrown into the fight for equality and justice to weaken us by keeping us separate. To me, this is about recognizing each other in the seemingly Other and standing together. We are undoubtedly stronger together.

Whiteness wants us to be distracted fighting each other because then we won't have as much in us to fight whiteness. We must reject being divided and conquered. It is in solidarity that we will find freedom.

What is crucial to realize, too, is that the ideology of white supremacy—the belief that the white race is superior to all other races—harms us all, including white people.

I think about the archetype of the spoiled child. He is constantly praised and catered to. He is given everything he wants, told he is the smartest, cutest, funniest, and most interesting person in the world. Doors—metaphorical and literal—are always opened for him. He can do no wrong.

How does the psyche of this child develop? Does he come to have a truly connected relationship to himself, to others, and to society? Does he ever come to know who he truly is if there is no room made for his imperfections, mistakes, and humanity?

And what, then, becomes his impact on those around him? How does he treat others? What does he expect of them? Does he bring love and care to his relationships and the spaces he is in?

* * *

I will never fully know what happened to my mother when she was pregnant with me and a few years later with my brother. But I can infer, based on my own experience as well as the numbers that plainly show that we mothers of color—we mothers of the global majority— are seen as less worthy, that it could not have been easy for her. I will never fully know what her mental health diagnoses were. I am not sure that she even got a clear answer herself, due to language barriers and cultural boundaries.

The weight of immigrant trauma and racial trauma alone can be too much for a person to bear. Adding also the trauma of becoming a mother for the first time—even with just the basic tasks of taking care of a baby let alone doing it without support. How did she do it? How do any of us?

I honestly think parents are superhuman.

It makes sense that my mother did not have the capacity to stay mentally well. Whether it was postpartum depression, bipolar disorder, anxiety, or a combination, whether it was purely due to a chemical imbalance or to all the aforementioned traumas, it manifested in her inability to mother. This, then, left me as her daughter untethered and uncared for, and seeking safety and control where I could.

3

Fed

Growing up, I always thought my mom was so beautiful. I loved seeing photos of her as a young college student, her dark brown hair long and straight, a style I've always been known for myself. She has large and light-colored eyes, something I always coveted. She was petite and naturally slim. She was sometimes compared to Princess Diana; even I could see a resemblance in their side profiles.

I admired everything about her—the thoughtfulness with which she put together her outfits and did her hair and makeup. I loved her so much, exactly as she was. All I wanted was to feel loved by her too. All children want and need this. Being on the receiving end of it now as a mother, I know that the unconditional love that a child has for their mother is incredibly deep and real. As mothers, we are their source of everything; we are where their very understanding of love begins.

So it was disorienting and upsetting that my mother rarely spoke kindly about herself. She was so self-critical, and she often blamed having had kids as the reason for her perceived ugliness: "I never had this fat on my stomach before having you kids. I hate this c-section scar. Look at all these white hairs from the stress you kids cause me. I need to go on a diet. I need to exercise, but I don't have any time for myself. I wish I could just get liposuction surgery. Mothers have to sacrifice everything!"

It took me years after having my first child to see the ways in which I was unconsciously repeating exactly what I had heard my mother say. I was obsessed with getting back to my pre-pregnancy weight and I never stopped talking about "those last ten pounds." I didn't even know what my exact weight had been when I got pregnant. I didn't own a scale and I understood that numbers fluctuate. But it didn't matter. I was always trying to be thinner and thinner and thinner so no number would ever have felt satisfying.

Pregnancy of course changed my body and I struggled to make peace with having needed an emergency C-section. I had lost the control I once had, the control I had depended on.

I became stuck in my inaccurate perceptions of myself, automatically playing my mom's tapes of self-criticism and my relationship to food became more disastrous than it had ever been.

With a C-section, you can't exercise for the first six weeks, so I turned to severe food restriction to help me lose the weight fast. As many moms can probably attest to, it doesn't take much effort to skip meals. It happens even if you don't want it to. Everything is just always so busy. I legitimately couldn't even remember if I had brushed my teeth on a given day. I got into an extremely unhealthy rhythm of eating poorly, if at all. Not eating affected my milk production, which I somehow did not understand would of course happen with low caloric intake. Not eating was also a major trigger for my anxiety and panic attacks.

I tortured myself by regularly trying to fit into clothes from when I was eighteen years old. If I'm being honest: I still have some of those clothes, including a pair of Seven low-rise bootcut jeans that I keep to use as a barometer of my bigness. I was back to my work teaching yoga and traveling for Nike just four months postpartum and at the start of every event, I practically hung my head in shame as I apologized to everyone for looking the way I did.

"I just had a baby, I'm still working on losing these last ten pounds."

I feel so sad for the new mom in me that was being battered by her inner critic. It destroyed my sense of self at the most fragile time of my life, when I needed the most support and love, including from within. And when I look back at photos, I cannot even see now what I thought I saw then.

I was only able to breastfeed my son for about three months. It had been a struggle from the very beginning. I had heard that breastfeeding burns a lot of calories and all I could think was, the less I ate, the even more calories I would burn. My thinking was so flawed, so damaging. What happened was that I produced so little milk to start that we had to feed him what little drops we could through a syringe. At the same time, I was so brainwashed into thinking formula was harmful that I ended up underfeeding him.

I felt like a failure that I couldn't produce enough milk to feed my baby. Wasn't this supposed to just happen naturally? But I now understand that I was not consuming enough. How could I feed my baby when I was not feeding myself?

All of these feelings of failure and unworthiness layered on top of each other, creating within me a deep hollowness. I felt like an imposter in all areas of my life—I had never felt more insecure in my job, I had no idea what I was doing as a mother, I was incredibly irritable with my husband, and I just despised myself. I pretended and masked when I needed to and I stewed in self-misery the rest of the time. I blamed motherhood for it all, because that's when I felt like I lost control.

Everything was unraveling. The combination of the hormonal changes, the new emotional extremes, and sleep deprivation meant that I simply could no longer live off of the adrenaline of weight loss and my tightly controlled persona. My body was revolting against the low blood sugar, the starvation, the self-abuse by way of crippling anxiety, insomnia, and panic attacks.

I spoke to Laura Iu, RD, CDN, CNSC, RYT, a registered dietician nutritionist and certified intuitive eating counselor who has worked at Weill Cornell & Columbia Medical Center of New York-Presbyterian Hospital, Mount Sinai Hospital, and NYU Langone Health. Iu affirmed my understanding of the connection between my anxiety and disordered eating: "I think even to your point about feeling anxious and having low blood sugar is that those symptoms overlap so much. There's such a parallel that it's really hard for someone to initially name or pick up or even recognize that, hey, maybe this isn't just about anxiety.

"This is actually because you're not eating enough. And our culture doesn't really push the narrative that you really need to nourish your body. You need to be eating adequately and regularly. As just a foundational piece, a foundational pillar to health. That's going to affect your mental health and emotional matters. Research studies support this. So if someone is quite restrictive on certain, foods, whether that's protein, carbs, or fat, it can increase their risk of anxiety and depression."

I wish I had had this information when I needed it. I wish I had been able to connect the dots between mental health, motherhood, and what it means to really nourish yourself.

Most days it would be around 4:00 p.m. that I would start feeling literally shaky. I always identified these shakes as an oncoming anxiety attack. I used to feel a similar wave of dis-ease every early evening during the newborn days, when I was barely holding things together, just trying to survive to the end of the day. It never occurred to me that maybe at least partly why I was feeling shaky and uneasy was because I had starved myself all day, but, why would I have thought this? It was how I had lived for most of my life until that point and it only became a problem once I became a mother.

* * *

The other day, I was out to brunch with my family. I had tried to order a Caesar Salad but after taking our order, the server returned to tell me that they were out. I took another look at the menu and saw that the Bibb Wedge Salad sounded similar enough and ordered it instead.

When the food arrived, the salad was placed in front of me. It was a wedge, alright. Literally just one big wedge of a bibb butterhead lettuce.

I was instantly transported to being ten years old at the kitchen table in my childhood home. I had recently decided I was vegetarian. I remember sitting alone at that table, eating half a head of lettuce, plain.

I had been horrified to learn about slaughterhouses. I have always felt a deep tenderness toward animals. As a young child, I joined both the World Wildlife Federation and the Nature Conservancy, sending in donations whenever I received birthday or New Year's money. Like most children, I hadn't known to question where my chicken nuggets or hamburgers had come from. As a mother, I've watched as my own children learned the truth and wondered how they could rationalize that another living being died so that they could consume it. My older one says a prayer of gratitude for the animal's soul; my little one pats whole chickens at the grocery store saying, "I love you little chicken."

Once I had connected the dots of how meat arrived on my plate, I could no longer eat it.

This was frustrating for my mother who cooked nearly all of the meals for the family. She was accustomed to cooking whatever she wanted, mostly Korean food, and aside from accepting that my younger brother needed the different foods on his plate to not touch each other, she made no special accommodations for any of us.

What I understand now as a parent is that nobody could force me to eat something I refused to eat. I had control of what I ate. It was perhaps the only thing I could control.

A lot of the time, I would just eat rice with seaweed or soy sauce and some of the vegetable 반찬—*banchan* (Korean side dishes)— my mom put on the table. I'd take any meat off of pizzas and opt for avocado and cucumber rolls if we went out for sushi. I have a fond and funny memory of sitting in a car with my grandmother who was visiting from Korea. Together, we finished an entire baguette while waiting for my mom to run errands.

Oh how I used to eat bread with such joy, and no guilt.

Sometimes, my mom would make something separate just for me. 콩자반—*kongjaban* (sweet and salty soybeans), 파전—*pajeon* (scallion pancake), and 두부—*dubu* (tofu) prepared in a variety of ways. I only understand in hindsight that all of this was my way of seeking signs of my mother's love.

*   *   *

I have a little scar on my stomach. When I was about nine years old, I was making ramen for my dad, my brother, and myself when for some reason, I picked up the pot while it was bubbling with boiling water. The scalding water splashed out and burned me through my clothes. I remember feeling shocked by the sudden pain.

My childhood was punctuated by seasons of my mom's depression. The more ramen I was making and the more empty Pizza Hut boxes there were stacked up on the kitchen counter, the worse and longer that particular bout of depression was. My mom would sometimes go weeks without changing out of her pale pink nightgown or opening her bedroom blinds. During these dark days, if she did get out of bed, she moved zombie-like through the house, no sign of vibrancy in her eyes.

And then one day, something would somehow shift. I would always wait in desperate hope for this shift. I would know the tide was turning when the kitchen would come back alive. The little tabletop stove would be back on the kitchen table for sizzling 찌개—*jjigaes* (stews) and 갈비—*kalbi* (marinated beef), the familiar smells of 된장—*doenjang* (fermented soybean paste) and 김치—*kimchi* (spicy fermented cabbage) filling the house again. The click of the rice cooker would tell us it was almost time for dinner.

My family never spoke about what it meant when my mom was cooking and when she wasn't cooking but we all understood the significance.

I watched the way my brother tried to connect with my mom through food. The two of them have always shared a similar palette. They both liked to eat foods I found too intense or too junky, like flaming hot Cheetos or the spiciest Korean *jjigaes*. Whenever my brother got in trouble, my mom would fly into a rage and banish him to his room. Awhile later, he would eventually reemerge and quietly make his way onto a bar stool across from my mom in the kitchen, who would still be fuming with anger. He would woefully say, "I'm kinda hungry . . ." and every single time, my mom would oblige. She would let out a hard sigh expressing disappointment and frustration at whatever trouble he had gotten himself into and then she would soften, ready to fulfill her duty to her youngest child.

I was grateful to my brother for his ability to restore and safeguard some peace in the house, if a little jealous that I could never seem to do the same. Being the firstborn daughter, though, I was expected to be able to make a meal for the family when needed. How could it possibly work for me to go to my mother, wide-eyed and hungry?

*   *   *

My eating habits continued becoming more and more restrictive. In addition to rejecting anything that came from an animal, I also started to obsess over food labels. This was the early 90s, when diet culture scared us all from consuming any fat.

In being difficult about food, I was subconsciously trying to force my mother's mental illness to stay away. I was sending the threatening message that if she were to disappear into her depression for weeks, I would have to survive on half heads of lettuce and then what would happen to me, her daughter, that she was supposed to take care of?

It was a deeply flawed and ill-conceived plan. The frightening oppression of my mom's cycles of depression inevitably would return. But the habit of my disordered eating only became more etched in. I was no longer eating the ramen and Pizza Hut that took the place of my mom's Korean home cooking. My brain had already categorized such foods as unhealthy and unsafe. I would end up subsisting on bread for breakfast, lettuce for lunch, and something like Reduced Fat Triscuits and an apple for dinner.

What I desperately needed was to be supported, parented, mothered. But my family was always too preoccupied with my mother to even notice that I needed help.

By the time I started practicing yoga in the diet culture-obsessed late 90s, I had become even more controlled about my eating. I was bouncing from one diet to another. No meat, no carbs, no sugar, no fat. I received constant praise for my discipline. What my body looked like felt like life or death. If I did not stay as thin as possible, I would lose it all.

Once I became a yoga teacher, I was obsessed with eating the bare minimum of foods that were least likely to cause bloat or otherwise be noticeable on my stomach through the lycra of Lululemon. Starchy carbs were obviously out alongside meat. Most days, I would get by on bananas, nuts, smoothies, and salads.

But with my full teaching schedule of up to twenty-five classes per week, I often found myself lightheaded and with low energy. My blood pressure was lower than it needed to be, but I tried to tell myself that maybe it was just from all the yoga and meditation I was doing. I was just *that* balanced and relaxed.

It was not at all sustainable to survive on handfuls of nuts. I didn't like the idea of eating a larger quantity of food, so I decided I needed to go back to eating meat. With a small quantity of meat, I could get a big hit of protein and therefore energy. I wasn't happy with the moral implication of eating meat again, but it was worth it if it meant I could continue avoiding carbs.

I would go through other phases of food limitations as I got deeper into my yoga life. At various points I returned to vegetarianism which morphed into veganism which further morphed into a raw diet based on eating "only what you could catch with your bare hands," a regimen a fellow teacher followed and shamed anyone who didn't do the same. I read that in eating anything that came from an animal, you were taking in their karma, and if an animal had been brutally slaughtered, you were consuming that energy of pain and suffering. I learned about the blood type diet and eating based on what your ancestors ate. I of course learned about the evils of gluten and took it as a moral victory every time I declined my once beloved bread basket.

The more I read about food, the more I wanted to read about it. It became an obsession. In lieu of consuming food, I consumed information about food. To this day I still own dozens of food and diet books. I didn't notice when the language of diet culture shifted to "clean eating" and I blindly jumped on that bandwagon. How could I eat in the most CLEAN way? How can I avoid all TOXINS?

There was an explosion of pressed juice companies and at-home masticators. I partook in it all, even becoming an ambassador for a pressed juice company. I did a seven or ten day juice cleanse four times a year for several years. I led "Detox Flow Yoga" workshops, teaching sequences that targeted the digestive organs, as if they would not be able to function without our literal manipulation of them.

I was a complete mess. I had so much information—much of it false and rooted in diet culture—swirling in my head that I would find myself paralyzed. What was safe to eat? A steak would be approved by Atkins and Paleo but too much red meat was bad for my heart and karmically cursed. Dairy was never a safe option for me as I was lactose-intolerant plus it supposedly worsened my eczema. Too much raw food seemed to give me stomachaches, perhaps incompatible with my Korean constitution that was traditionally built on fermented foods. Most prepared foods had hidden or not-so-hidden sugars or ingredients I could not pronounce, all of which were automatically out.

I would open the fridge and stand there, staring hopeless and defeated, unable to find anything that felt safe to eat. When you're trying to follow low or no carb *and* vegan *and* raw *and* gluten-free, there is hardly anything that is safe to eat. I read about great yogis who lived in caves and survived on oxygen and a few twigs and berries. I wished I could manifest into being like them.

I stuck to my list of "clean" foods and kept my quantities as small as possible. I was constantly restricting, which is a form of disordered eating, but I, and everyone around me just thought I was "disciplined."

* * *

I feel such grief and self-compassion as I come to understand my eating disorders more deeply. I was ultimately diagnosed with Body

Dysmorphic Disorder, Orthorexia, and Other Specified Feeding or Eating Disorder for my binge and restrict cycle. I was truly shocked, actually. I had truly thought I was just a health-conscious yogi who, if anything, needed to be *more* controlling. I couldn't face starting eating disorder therapy because all I could think was that the therapist was going to make me gain too much weight, so I ghosted her.

Diet culture is so normalized and as a society, we simply don't understand this. It was a struggle even trying to talk about it with a couple girlfriends. One waved it off and laughingly said, "ALL women have an eating disorder! I'm always on a diet!" Another friend, who has the genetically blessed measurements of a supermodel, could barely register what I had said, asking, "Wait, so, you're saying you should weigh MORE than you do?"

I felt ridiculous and quickly responded, "I know right, it totally doesn't make sense. If anything I definitely still have those last ten pounds to lose!"

I am sure that neither friend intended to be so invalidating. I think it speaks to our collective lack of understanding around eating disorders and mental health in general. Such as when we use phrases like "I'm so depressed" and "I wanted to kill myself!" in casual ways that undermine the true meaning of the words.

We also live in a society that praises and rewards extreme thinness and restrictive eating. I recently heard one of my former childhood idols, Jennifer Aniston, say, "Of course I indulge! I had **a** Dorito while waiting backstage." Watching *Friends* now, it's shocking to see how underweight nearly all the women on the show were. They're in their thirties and they probably don't weigh much more than my ten-year-old.

Of course, everyone has a right to their unique body shape and size—there is no space for body shaming at any size. Some people naturally have smaller bodies and some people naturally have bigger bodies; many of us fall somewhere between the two ends of the spectrum. Still, it cannot be denied that we have been inundated with representations of a certain body type as being the best, the most beautiful, the most desirable.

We have also grown up unconsciously accepting that there is a moral value ascribed to our physical size. "Wow, she must be so disciplined!" versus "Ooh, she's really let herself go." I don't need to specify which body type each of those statements bring to mind.

As well, it must be noted that these beauty and body standards are rooted in whiteness. Consider that the Body Mass Index (BMI), a tool still used for assessing health, has been deemed inaccurate, misleading, and racialized.

Dietician Iu explains, "the BMI was created based on statistical data from white Europeans, which we know doesn't account for the diversity of body types or genetic differences across other racial and ethnic groups especially here in the US. Since BMI doesn't consider muscle mass, bone density, or fat distribution, many people of color especially those with higher muscle mass, may be classified as 'overweight or obese'—which is pathologizing—despite being healthy.

"I think it's a big issue that BMI doesn't account for variations in body composition which can differ by race. For example, people of Asian descent are cited to have a higher body fat percentage at lower BMI levels. This actually led them to create a different set of BMI for Asians. It also contributes to eating disorders because people may see themselves pathologized. It is super harmful because they've doubled down on using BMI as a measure of health, rather than acknowledging that other factors can affect us. This all creates a ripple effect because we know health care bias and weight stigma exist."

The major learning here is that none of us deserve to be reduced to numbers, whether in weight, BMI, or calories. We have to ask ourselves who benefits when we put ourselves through diets?

What Iu does through her work is help people learn to eat intuitively so that you can figure out how to nourish your body with ease. Intuitive eating is the antidote to packaged diets, supplements, and exercise regimens. She says, "Diet culture is such a shapeshifter that so many people fall prey to the way diets will rebrand themselves as something else or talk about health or wellness. They are just adapting to the market and trying to speak to the most vulnerable. These companies will prey on people who have insecurities.

"I'm just here to give you another possibility to move away from that binary thinking. Some middle ground, some gray area in all of this, and then you can form your own decision around it. You have to figure out, is it true for you? Because if intermittent fasting is what's causing you so much distress, because you're so hungry that you're no longer grounded, you're irritated, you're dizzy, you're shaky, all those low blood sugar and anxiety symptoms. Is that really right for you?"

Intuitive eating is ultimately a decolonial, revolutionary praxis. Especially for women and mothers, it is a way for us to reclaim our power and to redefine our own standards of beauty, health, and wellness. We need to redefine our markers of health. Instead of shrinking ourselves to be as small as possible, what might happen if we consider the shine of our skin, the brightness of our eyes, the clarity of our cognition, the quality of our sleep, the sense of connectedness we have with our inner selves?

It took me finding out that I was pregnant with my daughter, a future woman and femme in this patriarchal society, to commit to finding food freedom. I no longer wanted to prioritize losing weight. I wanted to nourish myself so that I could nourish her. I wanted to embody self-acceptance, no matter my size. I never want my children to hear me demonize foods or criticize my perceived imperfections, no, I will do my best to exemplify the self-love that they—I, we—all deserve.

This has meant that I have been carrying more weight after my daughter than I did after my son. I still haven't "bounced back," but, what would I be trying to bounce back to anyway? Back to panic attacks and anxiety? No thank you!

Intuitive eating for us women of color is also an invitation back to the foods of our culture, an invitation to heal from experiences of racism.

Iu shares, "Only 5% of registered dieticians are Asian. The representation just isn't there. There's definitely a lack of understanding of just how important it is to have diversity in the field. So if you are trained with certain, namely Western, values, you're going to take that on and that is going to have a trickle effect when you are working with clients. In my experience, I was trained to think of Asian foods as being bad, unhealthy, and it went against everything I ever thought. So there I was, questioning, being told that when I go counsel my own patients, I'm supposed to tell them to cut out the sauces, cut out white rice? It's like asking someone to not be who they are. And it's such misinformation, that kale is better than *bok choy* or *galen*. I'm Chinese. We didn't grow up having salads. It's just not a thing. I think all of those messages are really harmful because someone can internalize these Western values around health. It can create a very shameful spiral around someone's health."

When I was caught in this shame spiral, I had never really considered how the imposition of white, Western beauty, body, and food standards were directly correlated to the harm I was causing myself. It makes sense, though: I knew that I could never be or even look white, but maybe I *could* achieve the thinness that was constantly being fed to us. So for more than half of my life, I ate in every way except for intuitively or aligned with my heritage.

As a child, I even rejected using chopsticks. I declared to my family, "I'm American! I am only using forks from now on!" I was just tired of being made fun of outside the home for being different. I didn't know to appreciate and be proud of being able to use chopsticks—it requires much more than it does to use a fork!

When I started to reclaim my Asian identity in college, I decided I wanted to use chopsticks again. I re-learned them incorrectly and to this day, mine still make an embarrassing x rather than stay side by side. I kind of like having this as a regular reminder of what happened when I rejected my roots. I won't let the bullying of others do that to me again. And it makes me more committed as a mother to raise my children—as they in turn raise me—to be proud of their mixed heritage.

It is because of my children that I have really started to reconnect to Korean foods. My son is obsessed with kimchi. He even eats kimchi at school—the cafeteria provides it! A lot of non-Korean kids eat kimchi. At home, he often requests that I add it onto his plate, no matter what cuisine we are eating, be it fried rice or tacos. I bought a new brand recently that turned out to be on the mild side. After tasting it, he asked if I could buy a different kind next time, "one with more spice, please!"

There is a fellow half-Korean classmate who Ryker is in awe of because he can take so much spice like it's nothing. "He says it's because we're Korean that we can take a lot of spice!" my son tells me with pride.

He chose 매운 새우깡—*mae-un saeukkang* (spicy shrimp crackers) as his after-school snack yesterday. He loved them so much that when he had to leave the table momentarily, he dramatically said to the bag, "I'm sorry I have to leave you, I will be right back!"

It is fascinating, and healing, to witness his joy over what to me had felt embarrassing as a child.

He asked this morning if we could order Korean takeout tonight. He loves the Korean foods I ate as a young child, before diet culture consumed me: 잡채—*japchae* (glass noodles), 멸치—*myulchi* (sautéed anchovies), and 돈까스—*donkkaseu* (the Korean take on the Japanese deep-fried pork cutlet) (because: colonization). Hilariously, no matter how many times I tell him that those crispy little fish are anchovies, he calls them sardines.

This past New Year's Day, I made for the first time a traditional Korean dish: 떡국—*dduk gook*—rice cake soup. Koreans always have *dduk gook* for New Year's as a way to usher in good luck. I loved *dduk gook* as a child. I can't remember the last time I've had it, as I stopped eating rice and rice cakes ages ago.

As I stood cooking at the stove, hoping I was making it correctly, I was overcome with emotion. I found myself was crying over *dduk gook*! It seemed so silly, but I know that it wasn't. It was so meaningful that I was cooking for my own kids a traditional Korean food that my mom made once made for me, when she was well enough, before I swore off meat, and eventually rice. Food being one of the only ways I knew my mom was still aware, still there . . . when I still felt hope of her mothering.

My daughter went on to have three servings of *dduk gook* that night. Words can't express the deep healing it brought me.

4

Bloodline

For most of my adulthood, I genuinely thought I had worked through any childhood trauma. In fact, I felt so fine about my past that I would not even have considered that I had been through any trauma. Nobody had ever used that word to describe what I had endured and survived. And besides, wasn't the main thing that I had indeed survived?

I never really talked to anyone about it so I both thought that maybe it was normal to have a mentally ill and abusive mother and that maybe it was so abnormal that I'd better not talk about it. I also believed that if I focused on the positive, I would manifest positivity—in my life and in my psyche. This mindset did seem to work for the most part . . . until I became a mother.

Whether it was due to hormonal changes or the sheer overwhelm of trying to keep a human alive, whatever control I thought I had fell apart. It was like motherhood was an unsolicited initiation into trauma. And once I stepped onto the path of excavation, it was as if that path had no end.

I have spent most of my life trying to make sense of my mother. As a child, I internalized her depression as being something I had caused and could therefore fix. As a teenager, I fled—literally, I ran away from home. As soon as I turned eighteen, I went to live with my best friend and her family for a couple months. She only lived a mile or two away, and I told my parents that that was what I was doing, so I guess it wasn't really running away. Still, my mom tried to stop me as I left, screaming at me and threatening me as I carried a brown paper grocery bag full of some clothes and toiletries. She tried to block me as I reached our front door, but I knew she couldn't physically stop me so I kept going. She grabbed chunks of my hair, as she had violently done hundreds of times before, but I forced my way out to my best friend who had been waiting for me in her car.

I eventually returned, knowing that I just needed to make it through a few more months before leaving for college. I told my dad that I needed us to go to family counseling in order for me to come home. I think we did one, maybe two sessions. I don't remember my mother saying anything. It was my way of trying to be heard, as well as warning them that our family was on someone's radar now. Kind of like calling child services, but a bit more subtle and strategic.

That was the last season of ever living with my parents. Once I moved to LA for college, I never even lived in the same city as them again. It was my way of protecting myself from my mother, though I don't know that I consciously understood it as such at the time. I was focused on creating my own life. I found yoga, built a teaching career, moved to Hong Kong and then to London, and got married. Not only did it feel like all my dreams were coming true, but it also felt like I had made peace with my childhood and with my unwell mother.

In actuality, I had done a brilliant job at repressing, coping, and dissociating, and motherhood was my initiation into unearthing the truth.

*   *   *

It is commonly understood that we tend to do unto others what was done unto us. But how far back does this relational connection go?

In 1966, Canadian psychiatrists Vivan Rakoff, MD, and John J. Sigal, PhD, first recognized the concept of generational trauma in their study "Concentration Camp Survival: A Pilot Study of Effects on the Second Generation," published in *The Canadian Journal of Psychiatry*. Their findings "suggest that there is a distinct possibility that the children of the concentration camp group may themselves rear disturbed children so that the wartime experience of the concentration camp parents may adversely affect the functioning of children generations removed."[1]

Generational trauma (also called transgenerational trauma or intergenerational trauma) is the idea that patterns of trauma response and maladaptive behaviors are carried through multiple generations. A simple example is repeating what was done to us to others: A child that was hit by her mother goes on to hit her child, despite having had the lived experience that this was morally wrong and damaging.

But what if you take the concept of generational trauma way back? What if you examine the trauma your ancestors may have experienced? Could you be impacted by experiences you did not directly have yourself?

Consider the fact that the egg that would eventually become you was already inside your mother's body when she was a fetus in her own mother's—your grandmother's—womb. In a 2021 *Psychology Today* article, licensed independent social worker-clinical practice Elizabeth Dixon wrote, "We know now that newborns don't enter into the world with a clean slate. Their emotional history begins even before they are conceived . . . [A] part of you, your mother, and your grandmother all shared the same biological environment . . . [Y]ou were exposed to the emotions and experiences of your grandmother even before you were conceived."[2]

It is widely accepted that when someone is pregnant, their mental and emotional states matter and could impact everything from the viability of the pregnancy to the physical and mental health of their unborn baby. Pregnant women are advised to keep their stress levels low. Mother and child are inextricably connected through the womb.

What generational trauma tells us is that we are also impacted by having existed as *cells* in our *grandmother's* womb.

As licensed clinical psychologist and parent evaluator Melanie English, PhD, told *Health* in 2022, "Generational trauma is trauma that isn't just experienced by one person—it extends from one generation to the next. It can be silent, covert, and undefined, surfacing through nuances and inadvertently taught or implied throughout someone's life from an early age onward."[3]

The same article goes on to quote child and adolescent psychiatrist and author Guyana DeSilva, MD: "Trauma affects genetic processes, leading to traumatic reactivity being weighted in populations who experience a great deal of trauma. . . . Being systematically exploited, enduring repeated and continual abuse, racism, and poverty are all traumatic enough to cause genetic changes. . . . People in countries that have endured years . . . of war may also have generational trauma."[4]

What Dr. DeSilva is saying is that the consequences of systemic oppression including racism and poverty as well as childhood abuse are deeply serious. These experiences are traumatic and change our actual genetic makeup. Generation trauma directly impacts our personhood.

Writer, doula, and mother Ashley Simpo shared with me how she feels the impact of generational trauma in her day-to-day life, especially in how she views labor—the labor not of childbirth but of work: "I think the way that we approach labor is definitely tied to what we've been taught about how we're supposed to feel about labor. I understand that the history of Black people in general dictates that

I'm going to be struggling with my relationship with labor. It's always going to feel like I have to detach from this idea that I have to be laboring all the time and this detachment is going to feel hard. I was recently sick and the hardest thing about it was allowing myself to rest. I was frustrated with myself because I knew in real time that this is a product of racism. I can't relax because relaxing or doing nothing is tied to the lazy slave trope that has passed through just a few generations. Slavery was not that long ago in terms of our families. So I understand that there are DNA patterns that literally exist in our bodies, that our ancestors unfortunately passed down to us. And we are constantly going to struggle with letting that go. And it does feel like it's a lot of work to do that."

Hearing and holding the stories of those that have been oppressed throughout history—especially a history not so long ago—matters because the impacts are being lived and felt in current time by our fellow human beings. I grew up learning that atrocities such as slavery, genocide, and war were mistakes of the past. That we as humanity had evolved past all of that. But now that I understand that those were all manipulated versions of the truth, I can make sense of the weight of injustice that has always lived in my bones and in my genes.

Additionally, it is important to consider that the impact of generational trauma is not only limited to large-scale, systemic traumas. Physician, psychiatrist, and *New York Times* bestselling author Dr. Daniel Amen explains that emotional trauma such as divorce, abandonment, incarceration, negative parenting behavior, or the early death of a family member can also have lasting consequences.[5]

Generational trauma can impact us all and the more we look to heal our individual selves, the more we can heal collectively.

The scientific research and understanding around generational trauma is a fairly new field of study. In an article titled "The Legacy of Trauma" published by the *American Psychological Association* in 2019,

Trauma Psychology president Diane Castillo, PhD, said, "[E]xcept for studies related mainly to the [Jewish] Holocaust, the field is still relatively young and has many unknowns. While trauma researchers have made great strides in understanding and treating single-episode present-life trauma, they are just beginning to explore the impact of intergenerational trauma and its expression."[6]

In yet the same article, Yael Danieli, PhD, added, "Continuing to explore intergenerational effects can help the field better understand and treat psychological pain at its roots. . . . Massive traumas like these affect people and societies in multidimensional ways. It behooves us to study this area as widely as possible, so we can learn from people's suffering and how to prevent it for future generations."[7]

That's why this research is so necessary: so we learn *how to prevent it for future generations.* Herein lies the hopeful idea that if *trauma* can be passed down through the generations, so, too, can *healing.* As Dixon wrote, "Fortunately, trauma survivors and their descendants can help to reduce the impact of generational trauma on future generations. Just as traumatic experiences can be passed down from one generation to the next, so can the capacity for overcoming the trauma and building resilience."

When we understand generational trauma in this greater context, one that *empowers* trauma sufferers and survivors, we can focus not just on the past but also proactively on the present, thereby influencing the future. Although we cannot control the past—what happened to us and to our ancestors—we do have agency right here and right now.

It's important to note that this sounds much simpler than it is. There are likely an array of complicated internal barriers and behavior patterns that make it difficult to access our genetic reservoir of resilience. But we can all start with acknowledgment followed by baby steps.

One example of how we can effect change is described in a 2018 study by *The Journal of Clinical Nursing*, which researched how to intervene in the intergenerational transmission of relational trauma within parent-infant relationships. Its primary finding was that "resolving parental trauma" and "actively supporting parent-infant attachment" were the key ways to prevent trauma transmission.[8]

To say it more simply, what the study is highlighting is the importance of a parent processing their own traumas as well as the importance of the bond between parent and infant.

If a major throughway of the transmission of trauma is from grandmother to mother to (grand)child, it is reasonable to think that the key to healing involves understanding what our mothers, grandmothers, and ancestors experienced and endured. This means that it is essential to have open communication within families and for children to feel seen, validated, and loved by their parents.

It also means that a mother's mental well-being is vital to her child's very livelihood. A mother's mental health influences the trajectory of her child's own mental health as well as their physical health; it is linked to the child's ability to survive and thrive, as it always has been since conception.

New scientific research is finding that our biology actually evolves based on the challenges our parents and ancestors experienced. In *Human Biochemistry*, Gerald Litwack, PhD, discusses noncoding DNA, which was formerly considered to be "junk DNA." Litwack explains, "Noncoding DNA makes up about 98.5% of the total DNA. While it was previously thought to have no function, newer information is beginning to shed light on the many functions of this mass of DNA. . . . It is . . . possible that noncoding DNA was used as a source of new genes needed for adaptation or for functions during evolution."[9]

In *It Didn't Start With You*, author Mark Wolynn further explains, "Noncoding DNA is known to be affected by environmental stressors, such as toxins and inadequate nutrition, as well as stressful emotions. The affected DNA transmits information that helps us prepare for life out of the womb by ensuring that we have the particular traits we'll need to adapt to our environment. According to Rachel Yehuda, epigenetic changes biologically prepare us to cope with the traumas that our parents experienced. In preparation for similar stressors, we're born with a specific set of tools to help us survive. . . . We're born with an intrinsic skill set—an 'environmental resilience,' as Yehuda calls it—that allows us to adapt to stressful situations."[10]

What all of these experts are emphasizing is that there is a way out literally built into our DNA. Our ancestors may have passed on a heavy load to us, and we may unknowingly have done the same to our own children, but each person's very biology has evolved to be able to handle it. The skill of resilience just needs some direction and practice like any other skill in life. It also needs your willpower and commitment to shatter cycles of harm.

I liken it to training any muscle in your body. You start where you are, but with consistent practice, you can increase strength, endurance, and flexibility. You can look at your epigenetic blueprint the same way. As Yehuda explained during an interview on the podcast *On Being*, "there is a wisdom in our body . . . . [O]ne of the studies that we published . . . showed that some epigenetic changes occur in response to psychotherapy. If we're saying that environmental circumstances can create one kind of change, a different environmental circumstance creates another kind of change, that's very empowering."[11]

Although epigenetics is well beyond the scope of this book, the basic idea is that what happened to your parents, grandparents, and ancestors informs and impacts your very biology, your genetic predispositions, and your own emotional and psychological landscape. But the effects of these environmental circumstances are not immutable or permanent.

Consider also that future generations tend to have many advantages over preceding generations: for example, children growing taller than their parents and the average lifespan increasing. Even as trauma is passed down, future generations have access to what previous generations don't: the potential skills and tools to survive and overcome. Each subsequent generation is then theoretically better equipped to heal, to be a cycle breaker. We are not destined to suffer and we do not have to pass our suffering down.

Therapist, author, and advice columnist for *The Washington Post*, Sahaj Kaur Kohli provides important context around the role of the cycle breaker in our interview: "It's a privilege to even be a cycle breaker. I don't think you need to have certain privileges to be a cycle breaker, but I do think you need to have the privilege of self-awareness and not being in survival mode to be able to even identify that something needs to be broken. We know more now than we ever did about intergenerational trauma. We're talking about these things more and more, we're able to understand that there are macro and collective experiences, whether it's colonization or war or genocide and how our ancestors endured those. Even if we don't have access to the very people who did experience those, we can know through history books what that was like and think about how that might have impacted them.

"For us children of immigrants, for example, I don't have access to my grandparents. They're no longer alive. When they were alive, I didn't have the wherewithal to even know to ask them some questions. And so I have done my own research, read books on the partition of India in 1947, and come to understand that my grandparents were refugees who had to cross the border with very little. I've learned from my parents who have gone back to what is now Pakistan, where my families on both sides are originally from, prior to the partition. I have heard stories of people who knew our families. And that's how I'm gaining access to my family history. Even though I can't talk to my ancestors, I'm learning. I'm able to maybe make assumptions and to also theorize what my grandparents went through. I wonder what that was like for them. I wonder what they learned because of these experiences. And naturally, everyone learns skills to cope with pain and trauma. I knew from when my grandmother was alive that she was very forward thinking, didn't want to talk about the past, and was very avoidant if I did ask any questions. I can surmise that that led my mom to learn emotional suppression, which then I can make the connection to why I have always felt like my emotions were bad or too much."

There is so much to be gained from learning about our family's histories in whatever way we can. For those of us who don't have access to any living blood relatives, we can research the lands and cultures that we come from. We can put ourselves into the shoes of those who experienced traumatic events. We can write the stories that we ourselves need to hear.

And as we identify the traumas we may have inherited, so too must we seek to discover the tools of resistance that were bequeathed to us. Kohli reminds us, "We don't just inherit trauma and fears and pain. We also inherit dreams. We inherit resilience. We inherit adaptability, traditions, community building skills, humor, stories. We inherit so much more. And I think a part of addressing intergenerational trauma is also addressing intergenerational strength and all that help us feel connected to our ancestry, to our history, to our roots, knowing that we can persevere and endure and change, on a macro scale but also on a micro scale."

I am starting to understand that generational trauma is so much more than the baseline of my mental health challenges. Maybe it's more like a treasure hunt—what gifts have my grandparents, ancestors, and Korean history left for me to discover?

* * *

I wish I had asked my grandparents so many more questions when they were still alive.

Why did they know how to speak Japanese?

Why did Halabuji join the army?

What was daily life like in the wake of war?

How are things different now, decades later?

Do you know what happened to your family who remained in the North?

When I think about my grandparents, I think mostly about my maternal side. I always felt more relaxed around them. There seemed to be more formality expected around my paternal grandparents. I could also sense my parents' timidness when we went to visit my dad's side.

All four of my grandparents lived in South Korea so I mostly only got to see them on our summerlong visits back to the motherland. My maternal grandparents would occasionally come and see us in California and when they did, they sometimes stayed for weeks.

I always loved having them around. I loved eating bread with my Halmuni, and sitting near my Halabuji as he watched and chuckled at endless reruns of *The A Team,* a military show that was lighthearted and comedic. I think he must have been seeking his own healing from his experience of war.

My grandparents' presence seemed to keep my mom's depression at bay, whether by actually helping her feel more supported or because she felt like she had to pretend like everything was okay when they were visiting. Things just felt more normal when they were around.

While I do speak Korean, my vocabulary is limited. I can make small talk and order food, but I can't understand the news or talk about my feelings with any depth. Although, even if I could talk about my feelings in Korean, I don't know that this is something I ever would have done, being that such touchy feely conversation is outside of our cultural norms.

Still, there was a closeness I felt with my grandparents—a safety, even, in knowing that my mom would not dare be abusive to me in front of them. As much as she demanded obedience from me, she had her own daughterly duties to her parents.

There was a palpable sense of reverence for my Halabuji from everyone who was around him. As children, we had heard stories about him having been in the army. I didn't really know the specifics of what that had entailed, but it made me think that my Halabuji was brave, strong—a hero. That's why I kept it between him and me when I caught him sneaking cigarettes in the bathroom.

He had forgotten to lock the door once and I walked in to find him blowing smoke into the ceiling vent. He looked at me and put his index finger to his mouth with a glint in his eye. I was delighted to get to have a secret of his to hold.

*　*　*

The story of my grandparents' escape from the North to the South has always been family lore.

Exact dates were never given, but the official timeline of the Korean War is June 25, 1950—July 27, 1953. In the story, my eldest aunt, who was born in 1950, was an infant and my grandmother was pregnant with my mother, who would be born in April 1952.

The story goes: My Halmuni and Halabuji fled south on foot, facing danger along the way. My Halabuji was a 소장—*So Jang* (Major

General) in the army, and he was wanted by the enemy. They were held at gunpoint, my Halmuni lost her shoes and begged for her daughter and her unborn child to be spared. They all survived. Eventually, my mother and three additional children were born, and everyone lived happily ever after.

That's how my child's mind neatly packaged the story anyway.

My first memories of visiting them in Seoul were nothing out of the ordinary. They lived in a modest apartment building, no different from most of the high-rises throughout the city. They were healthy, able-bodied, and looked happy. I didn't know to question what life had been like for them after the war "ended." I didn't even know to try to imagine what life could have been like for them.

* * *

We all understand the basic fact that genes are shared within biological families. We see this in the shared physical traits among biological family members. There is also often a palpable sense of connection and *familiarity* among people who are related. I see it when our children are with their cousins: an instant, effortless rapport even without having seen one another for years. Blood recognizes blood.

I have a cousin in Korea who I am very close to despite our lifelong geographical distance. She is my mom's sister's daughter, so we have the same maternal grandmother, the same Halmuni. My cousin and I became mothers around the same time and we both experienced the ground shaking, identity collapsing changes that motherhood can bring. We both found ourselves in postpartum depression with symptoms we had seen in our mothers: we were anxious, we felt hopeless, we worried we'd made a mistake in having a child. We were both terrified that we were doomed to become like our moms.

It can feel alarming to recognize that genes of mental illness run in your family. This must be the best possible explanation as to how my cousin and her mother, living on the other side of the world, are playing out such a similar narrative to my mother and me. And aren't we stuck with the genes that we're born with? I certainly can't alter my physical genetic reality—my eyes are the color that they are—so how can I possibly posit that I could alter my mental-emotional genetic profile?

What we all have to remember is that genes of trauma are not our whole story. Yes, we are influenced by generational trauma but we have to remember that we are not the exact same person as our mothers, as our ancestors. This is a complex but equally promising perspective on why we may be experiencing the disorders, symptoms, pain, and difficulties that we do. It brings me relief to think that it is not a genetic guarantee that I will repeat my mother's mistakes and forever relive my family's traumas. Rather than a life sentence, maybe it is an opportunity to burn through the karma of our bloodlines.

I think about the fact that my mother was born during the Korean War. I think of my grandmother's fear and terror, raising children in such a threatening time. How she and my grandfather ran for their lives and for the lives of their babies. I can't help but connect the dots to my panic attacks that would seemingly come out of nowhere, filling me with alarm and fear, making me feel the need to run for my life.

I think about my grandfather losing his parents and siblings to what would become North Korea. An entire lineage lost to us forever.

I think about how the war never ended. We Koreans continue to be a divided people still technically at war.

How could we, my own family as well as Koreans collectively, not be negatively impacted by this: an unfinished, mass-scale trauma that happened in our parents' lifetime, only a few decades ago?

According to my therapist of eight years, Alan Cohen, LCSW, LP, past traumas of older generations perpetuate into the present when handled in one of two main ways. Considering once again families who survived the Jewish Holocaust, on one end of the spectrum is the family that never stops talking about the Holocaust. The children in this family live in the trauma of the Holocaust because the stories of horror, loss, fear, and death are repeated, explicitly brought into daily life. On the other end of the spectrum is the family that never talks about the Holocaust. The children in this family also live in the trauma of the Holocaust through the attitudes, behavior, body language, and emotional patterns of their parents. This latter example may have a more damaging effect as it can cause children to question their own intuition, their sense that they are not being told the truth.

My family, as is the case with many Asian cultures, is of that latter camp of never talking about things. Whether my parents' intention was to protect us or if it never even occurred to them to do things differently from what had been done to them, I can firmly attest to the fact that it only made things worse for my brother and me. The blanks that are left by that which is not explicitly said can feel even more frightening than the truth because our imagination knows no bounds and we can endlessly create worst-case scenarios in our minds. Whereas when you're told the truth, even a hard, heartbreaking truth, there is often a deeply reassuring resonance, a confirmation of that which feels real. We all feel this, perhaps children most of all, with their yet untainted connection to their intuition, their inner knowing of what feels true and right in their literal bodies.

*   *   *

In thinking about all that we genetically inherit, I'm struck by a Korean word, concept, and state of beingness: 한—*Han.*

It is said that there is no exact translation for *Han* into English. This disconnect makes sense when you consider that the word seeks to express the experience of being oppressed and English is the oppressor's—or colonizer's—language. English is the language imposed on people whose lands were occupied, stolen, and colonized by English-speaking nations including Britain and the United States.

Korea has a long history of oppression, most notably in recent history with the Japanese occupation of 1910–45. The end of Japanese occupation was also the beginning of a divided Korea, with the United States suggesting two occupation zones: the Unites States would occupy the South and the Soviet Union would occupy the North.

The Korean War followed a few years later, and South Korea (aka the Republic of Korea) continues to be militarily occupied by the United States. The two countries signed the Mutual Defense Treaty in 1953, establishing extensive US military presence in Korea. The United States continues to have wartime operational control of Korea, as reported in March 2025 by Lee Hyo-jin in The Korea Times.[12] According to the US Department of Defense, there are currently 28,500 US service personnel station in South Korea.[13]

I used to think that the past is in the past. We read about it in history books and hear stories from family members. The concept of *Han* gives us a clue that perhaps the impact of the past is actually very present in our very selves.

In Arabic, there is a similar word: قهر—*qaher*. Although the literal translation is simply "anger," similar to *Han*, *qaher* holds the multilayered weight of anger, grief, and suffering. Psychotherapist, author, and mother Lena Derhally is a diasporic Palestinian American whose grandparents were expelled from their homeland of Bethlehem in 1948—incidentally the same year that Korea was officially divided. Derhally says, "*Qaher* is used when someone is mistreated, abused, or oppressed. It's difficult to directly translate it to English."

Language seeks to make meaning of what we experience, ever evolving in an attempt to most accurately describe that which can sometimes feel impossible to describe. This is always the work of artists, of poets and painters and composers, to capture the threshold of human experience. That two such similar words exist in two such disparate languages feels nothing short of a divine signpost. What answers might we find about the impact of our bloodlines and ancestral history on our health and well-being? What other languages might hold similar clues to our healing?

For Koreans, the residue of occupation and a war that never ended remains visceral, as real as the thirty-eighth parallel dividing our land and separating our people—our literal kin with a shared lineage. The truth of this cuts into my soul with an immediacy that used to confound me—I was born decades after the Korean War, after all— until I came to understand *Han*.

Han encompasses the sacred emotions of rage, despair, regret, sorrow, grief, and so much more. I believe *Han* lives in my cellular memory. I believe *Han* is the language of my soul, my spirit, my ancestors, my land. I believe *Han* is an energy that insists on being activated and reckoned with. I believe that everyone has a version, an interpretation of this energy.

I believe *Han* manifests as generational trauma, cycles of abuse, and mental illness when left uninvestigated.

I also believe that when *Han* is tethered to a purpose rooted in healing, love, and truth, an alchemy happens.

I believe that it is *Han*—knowing the stories and history that we come from—that ultimately sets us free.

* * *

My cousin expressed to me that while she feels heavy with the inherited burden laid upon us by our family history, she also derives strength from understanding more about how trauma moves through generations. She told me, "I know I have to do something. I have to stop whatever this is from getting to my kids."

I, too, am committed to doing better than was done to me. While I can hold compassion for the pain my mother has endured, and the pain of all of our bloodline before her, I cannot excuse the harm she caused me as a child. That would make it excusable for me to do the same to my children. It is only by holding her accountable for her choices that I can hold myself accountable for mine. And I want to be accountable for my choices. It means that I can have freedom from my genetic blueprint. It means that I have agency. It means that I can be a cycle breaker.

5

Village

"It takes a village," we hear over and over again. Mothers, especially, know the truth of this saying.

In American society—and throughout the West—we are rewarded for being independent. And not only independent, but the best, #1, the winner. So much of our culture is rooted in award ceremonies and competitions, from the Oscars to the Olympics. We are judged and ranked by our ability to be better than each other.

Some of the most American of values include ambition, persistence, chasing the dream, achievements, and accolades. How much can you do? How much can you earn? How impressive is your CV?

What results is hyperindividualism, which *The Oxford Review* describes as "an extreme focus on personal autonomy, self-reliance, and independence, often at the expense of community, social responsibility, and collective well-being. It is characterized by the prioritization of personal success and interests over group or societal needs."[1]

What this leaves out is a sense of community. Even when you experience being on a team, it can often still be in the context of competing against another team, be it in beating another team in a sport or in trying to win an account at work.

This obsession with independence and individualism leads to particularly harmful consequences for women. Because we live in a patriarchal society, rife with unequal wages and opportunities where 46 percent of women globally (64 percent of women in America) don't feel safe when walking alone at night,[2] women are already working harder than men to simply exist. The patriarchy has designated us as the inferior gender, which doesn't make sense considering we are the ones that are able to create and sustain literal life with our bodies.

Because this patriarchal society manufactures scarcity for women, we often end up in competition—rather than in community—with each other. Somewhere along the line, we get the message that asking for help or not looking perfectly put together signifies weakness, and so we end up living inauthentically, fraudulently even. And we influence other women to do the same, perpetuating the cycle of harm to our very selves.

Consider the idea of "having it all." It typically applies to a woman's ability to have a career, a partner, a house, AND BE A MOM. Mothers are the ones asked, "How do you do it all?" whereas fathers being home to look after their own children might be considered to be "babysitting." A majority of mothers - 71.7 percent of mothers work outside of the home while also being the primary caretaker[3] / executive assistant / chef / housekeeper / tutor, and more, to their children.

Even the term—*working mother*—signifies that we live in a patriarchy. Have you ever heard of a man with children being called a working father?

When I was pregnant with my first, I was dead set on doing it all by myself. I had no access to an organic village but it also did not even occur to me to look into hiring any sort of help. I just knew I could do it all. I had done most everything else by myself throughout my life. I had been a super responsible child—whether that was due to my innate personality or borne of necessity (probably both). I moved away for college, always had jobs, paid my bills, and lived in different countries. I had navigated a variety of cultures, languages, work environments, and social circles. I had never been able to rely on my mentally ill mother for life advice, so it was never an expectation that I would be able to rely on her when I was becoming a mother myself. I had always figured things out on my own . . . why would motherhood be any different?

Being in London during my first pregnancy, I had the added isolation from any long-term friends. Everyone in my day-to-day life was relatively new: yoga teacher colleagues or family and friends I'd met through my husband. I hadn't yet reached the depth of trust with anyone aside from my husband, the kind of trust that can only come with time.

In hindsight, I can see that I was putting on a brave face for myself because I didn't feel like I had any other choice. I looked at my life, my world at the time, and other than my husband, I couldn't see anyone with whom I could be my weakest, ugliest, saddest, scared self. Perhaps this had as much to do with my location in geography as it did my repression of trauma, which I would only become aware of in the months and years following my son's birth.

My belief and insistence that I would be *just fine* doing it all by myself was perhaps most apparent in what I said to my yoga students and clients. A large part of my work was traveling to teach events and lead trainings, whether for Nike or at independent yoga studios. I had a residency at a studio in Singapore, where I led three-week teacher trainings every few months. I would fly from London to Singapore, live in a random rented room, and teach twelve-hour days, six days a week.

When I was planning my maternity leave, which at the time was a very reasonable nine months paid, with my job being protected for up to a year (though all my employers and clients were amenable to longer), I told everyone I expected to be back in a month. The naivete! I would teach up until a week before my due date and planned to be back to my regular schedule a month after having the baby. I even had my next Singapore trip scheduled for less than four months postpartum.

I was unable to even conceive of what I needed to be planning for. I had not asked myself: Who was going to look after the baby while I was teaching? What if he needed feeding? Changing? Rocking? What if he cried? Screamed? All of the above?

My nonchalance was unhinged. "It will be fine," I told myself, willing it to be true because I could not handle the enormity of what it would mean if it weren't true.

My two sisters-in-law in London urged me to join my neighborhood "mums" group. The local council (i.e., town hall) brings together groups of expecting mothers based on post code and due date. I looked into it, but I never signed up. Partly because I didn't think I needed anyone else, but I now understand that it was also partly because I didn't think I would fit in. I didn't think that it would necessarily be a safe space for me as an Asian American MOM, not mum. I was so accustomed to being an outsider and feeling rejected that I often preemptively rejected myself from a potentially uncomfortable situation.

I wildly underestimated what was ahead. Until you become a mother, you simply cannot understand how maddening the basic logistics of motherhood are.

Because—how hard could it be? Right??

Well.

Giving birth, for starters, is a massive ordeal. I do not think we acknowledge this enough. And this is true whether you felt totally supported and happy with your birth or you felt that your birth was traumatic. A HUMAN WHO DID NOT PREVIOUSLY EXIST, EXISTS NOW.

Can we marinate on the hugeness of this fact?

I don't care if billions of women have given birth throughout human history and that 367,000 babies were born each day in 2023 alone (according to UNICEF).[4] Each baby being born is a huge deal and at the most basic level brings many operational life changes.

Nothing is the same. And I mean literally.

It's not as simple to just do what you want or need to when you want or need to. Keeping your baby alive is your new priority and purpose, and you are learning on the job while you are likely being cried on, vomited on, or slept on while you yourself probably also need to cry, vomit, and sleep.

It's hard to make yourself food, to remember to eat it, to have your coffee or tea hot (while worrying is it okay to have coffee or tea if you're breastfeeding), or to drink enough water. The basics of daily hygiene that you once took for granted are no longer guaranteed. Leaving the house has never been more complicated or burdensome . . . it's like packing a Go Bag every single time for all of the just-in case-scenarios. An extra pacifier in case I drop or God forbid lose this one. Extra clothes in case of blowouts or sudden temperature changes. Formula, bottles, keep warm and keep cold packs, diapers—so many diapers— wet wipes—how did we live before always having wet wipes on hand?

And what kind of transportation makes the most sense? A stroller is convenient to hold all the aforementioned items but what if I need to take stairs in and out of train stations or brownstones?

The mental labor alone is unlike anything I had experienced before, and I found myself tackling most of it on my own on most days, as my husband only had a paltry two weeks of paternity leave.

The more overwhelmed I felt, the more desperately I clung to the false mantra that it would all be fine. I couldn't admit that I needed support because where would that support come from? Who could I call? Who could I rely on?

I did eventually find fellow moms through friends, which I liked because it felt more organic than joining the local mums group. There were a couple new mothers at my husband's work who I got to know, and our shared commiseration about the incessant needs of our newborns proved to be a lifeline. Mostly, I relied on my phone to soften the isolation that I felt. I texted my girlfriends back in the United States, googled whatever I was uncertain about as a new mother (which was basically everything), and followed momfluencers. A lot of moms create a makeshift digital village in this way. The thought is that it's better than total isolation, but what we really need is each other, in person, in real life.

Mother and psychiatrist Pyravin Abbasova shared, "I feel like the biggest blessing is other women in your life. Because as much as you love your partner, physiologically he's not going to be able to relate to you and really understand what you go through. Ultimately your support, if you don't have a mother, if you don't have family members, is in a community of women. To me, my biggest help were always women that I met organically. I tried to join mom groups but they didn't often work for me. So it was randomly meeting women, like in a park. You just see some mom who your energy clicks with. You understand that other moms feel the way you do. It's so natural for us to want to be with each other, to want to flock together. It's such a natural instinct. Don't be afraid to put yourself out there and try to talk to a mom. You might discover that she's functioning on the same level of dysfunction as you are."

The *same level of dysfunction* is so real. When you really see that you're not the only one struggling, it softens the sting of the struggle. With other mothers you can commiserate and even laugh. You can grow into motherhood together.

I loved Dr. Abbasova's story of how she met one of her dearest mom friends: "I was living in an apartment complex with my first baby and I remember seeing another young mom in the neighborhood. I would notice her walking by with a stroller. She lived a couple of buildings down and she put a note in everyone's mailbox. The note said, 'I'm a stay at home mom. I have a baby. If you also have a baby, if you want to hang out, how about we meet at the park?' And I decided to show up. I was the only one who showed up but I'm so glad I did because we became friends.

"Sometimes you have to make this kind of effort because we can all live in our own homes and apartments and never talk to each other. But it's very validating when you talk to another mother and you realize you are experiencing the same things. You feel so much better because of the connection."

It can be daunting to seek new friendships in adulthood, and especially when you're just starting to figure out who you are in your new role as a mother. It's also likely to be a hit-and-miss process, not unlike dating. But the joy of connection and community is as essential as it is validating. Some mothers are lucky to have built-in villages comprised of relatives and childhood friends. For those of us that don't, we can—and must—build our own.

In addition to cultivating relationships with other mothers, we need people in our lives who are there to support and advocate for us.

Writer and doula Ashley Simpo shares: "I did not inherently think of motherhood as something you need a team for. I did not inherently think about how to set up a village around my baby or that I was going to need aunts and uncles to show up. I got some really good advice from a woman that contributed to a book I was editing, about parenthood in the first year. She doesn't have any children of her own, but she's an aunt to her siblings' kids. And she told me that you have to hand the baby over early. You have to have somebody else bathe

the baby and dress the baby and let them bond with other people so that those relationships can start to form. We do inherit this idea that we have to do it by ourselves. And that's the problem. I think that when you step back from that, it really changes things. It's hard to do, though."

What Simpo is saying is completely opposite to the mindset I went into motherhood with. It's not about proving I can do it all alone—it's about learning to rely on others. It's about expanding both your and your baby's world. It's about rooting into Indigenous, tribal ways, back when it was the norm for multiple generations to live together.

Realizing this need to approach pregnancy, birth, and motherhood differently from what mainstream modern life sets us up for is what inspired Simpo to start looking into how she could help other mothers: "It began through seeing my sister go through it, then researching and reading a lot of books. I was taking classes. I was doing all of these different things just to understand how to have a birth without being messed with by anybody. My curiosity started there and then every other friend who got pregnant after that would just reach out to me and say, do you have any advice? What should I do? Do you know a doula or a midwife? And so the resource sharing part of it started a long time ago for me. And I think that's something that mothers do naturally with each other."

This sharing of resources, experiences, and wisdom is what happens in the context of a village. Mothers need other mothers who are in similar phases of motherhood to relate to, mothers who have more experience to learn from, and even mothers who are newer to bring along because in being able to be the one that helps others, we benefit too. When we can feel like we have helped someone else, we feel useful and valuable, and this builds confidence. This is all built into the village—the reciprocity of roles and relationships.

*   *   *

Today, more than ten years into my motherhood, I finally feel like I have the makings of a village. It has never been built in for our family, as all of our relatives live thousands of miles away, mine to the west and my husband's over the pond to the east.

My older one has friends from school in the neighborhood who we have now known for several years. I can send him off on his own from our home to theirs, knowing there are caring parents on the other side. We all rely on each other to help with last minute pick ups and drop offs. Our homes are open to each others' kids.

My younger one is still little at four years old, so she's not quite ready to be walking through the streets of Brooklyn on her own yet, but she has grown up in the company of her older brother's friends and their families. They all look out for her at playdates and parties. Her world is not confined to just one caretaker at home, and I can see the expansive impact this has on her developing psyche and personality.

A friend of mine recently celebrated her birthday with a weekend of festivities. She rented a brownstone so that out-of-town friends could have the option to all stay together. I brought my daughter with me to the house on the first day and my friends—who aren't parents themselves—immediately and instinctively welcomed her in.

It was so beautiful to see that my daughter could just sense that she was cared for and safe in this new environment. And my friends stepped in playing games and making art with her, knowing that I would appreciate the reprieve from mothering. At first, I kept checking in, "Are you okay with her? Do you want me to take over? Do you need me to bring you anything?" It just felt so foreign to experience such an organic, easeful moment of me being taken care of as a mother.

As well, we are fortunate to have the financial privilege of hiring a weekly babysitter for date night, but hired help feels different because it is ultimately transactional. And while transactional does not mean without care and connection, it is not the same as having a village.

*   *   *

In collectivist cultures including Asian, Latin, and Native, a new mother is never expected to tackle her foray into motherhood on her own. In many of these cultures, there is a postpartum confinement period of around forty days, where the mother is centered and supported, typically by other women.

According to La Leche League GB, an organization providing breastfeeding support in Great Britain, "This forty-day period crops up again and again, from India to Mexico to Palestine, although a Korean mother describes how 'at least 21 days is good; 30 days is even better; even up to 100 days if possible.' . . . One almost universal aspect of postpartum traditions is that the new mother must rest."[5]

I spoke to my sister-in-law, a native Korean who had her first two children in Seoul, South Korea. She told me about 산후조리—*Sanhujori*, the sacred period of twenty-one days of postpartum healing and recovery for mothers: "*Sanhujori* is a period of time where you don't go outside, you take care of your body, and you stay warm. You eat 미역국—*miyukgook* (seaweed soup) every day. Traditionally, this was all done by someone like your mom or your grandmother. After the financial crisis of 2008, *sanhujori* centers—조리원—*joriwon*— became more popular, which is where I went for my first baby. Then for my second baby, I hired a *Sanhujori emo* (aunt) who came to our home, since you can't have any other kids with you at the center."

My sister-in-law also shared that several of her friends who don't live in Korea have even traveled to Korea to be able to stay at a *sanhujori* center, and for those who can't travel, there are Korean midwives offering this *sanhujori* support out of their own homes.

Even the *New York Times* has covered these maternity centers, as Lauretta Charlton reports: "Sleep is just one of the luxuries provided by South Korea's postpartum care centers. Fresh meals are delivered three times a day, and there are facials, massages, and child-care classes. Nurses watch over the babies around the clock. Staying at a *joriwon* can cost from a few thousand to tens of thousands of dollars. Insurance does not cover the fees, but they can be subsidized by the government through a stipend meant to encourage more families to have babies."[6]

Charlton continues, "Now eight out of 10 South Korean mothers go to a *joriwon* after giving birth. . . . Part of the appeal of booking a *joriwon* is the chance to spend time with other first-time moms who have children of the same age."[7]

Whether or not a new mother receives support from her own family or by affording a stay at a *joriwon*, the cultural understanding is clear: the focus on the mother's recovery is essential. Whereas I wanted to jump back into my old life, treating my new role as mother as but an addendum to my existing identity, my Korean kin have known to safeguard their healing with the help of elders and professionals. I can't help but think that a deep part of me that expected and needed this care must have felt so abandoned.

*   *   *

In America, isolation as a new mother is the cultural norm. A Harvard study called *Loneliness in America* found that "51% of mothers with young children feel 'serious loneliness.'" This "miserable degree of loneliness" indicated "feeling lonely 'frequently' or 'almost all the time or all the time.'"[8]

The report continued, "The cost of loneliness is high. Loneliness is linked to early mortality and a wide array of serious physical and emotional problems, including depression, anxiety, heart disease, substance abuse, and domestic abuse."

The epidemic of loneliness is a health crisis. With mothers of young children being disproportionately impacted, the very foundation of the family and home life is at risk. The mental and emotional weight alone can understandably become too much to bear.

What's more: Mothers are expected to bounce back—there is pride in getting your body back—in essentially erasing the fact that you have given birth. I'll never forget seeing a mom from my son's preschool running down the street three days after delivery. When I expressed concern, she insisted that she was fine—*great*, even.

*   *   *

I wish I could go back in time to my just-pregnant self and tell her: You don't have to do this by yourself. You're not supposed to do this by yourself.

Even with a partner in my husband, we were still left to divide and conquer our time so that we were much more frequently 1:1 with our baby than 2:1 together as three. Still, the case for a village asks for more than just the three of us, more than the nuclear family.

The nuclear family is defined by the *Encyclopaedia Britannica* as "a group of people who are united by ties of partnership and parenthood and consisting of a pair of adults and their socially recognized children. Typically, but not always, the adults in a nuclear family are married. Although such couples are most often a man and a woman, the definition of the nuclear family has expanded with the advent of same-sex marriage. Children in a nuclear family may be the couple's biological or adopted offspring. Thus defined, the nuclear family was once widely held to be the most basic and universal form of social organization."[9]

Without being able to pinpoint exactly when or how I learned about the nuclear family, I know I was very young when I started holding the idea of this dream, which I now see is reinforced everywhere in children's media. A mom, a dad, 2.5 children, a golden retriever, and of course a white picket fence. I didn't know to think of this in the context of capitalism or hyperindividualism. But the truth is this: The more we adhere to the model of the nuclear family, the more we end up feeding the system of capitalism. We will need to become laborers, we will probably opt for mortgages and other loans, we will put our children into the systems of education, healthcare, and perhaps also opt into religion and the military.

I recently rewatched the 1999 film *The Matrix*. Doing so in 2025 is quite jarring. The film is ultimately an allegory of humans as capital. The character Morpheus distills the message in one quick moment of holding a battery up to camera. Humans have been reduced to being used as batteries. The antagonist in the story is AI, which is certainly literally believable and eerily relevant at this current moment in our history, but we can also look at AI in the film as a characterization of capitalism.

In *The Matrix*, human beings are bred solely for the purpose of powering AI (or being a cog of capitalism), devoid of all that makes us human—our longing, our creativity, our thoughts. Perhaps most of all robbed of our love—our *need*—for each other, for connection. Each individual is literally confined to their own pod, kept completely separate from others.

Similarly, in the nuclear family, each family unit is effectively in their own pod. Separated, physically, from our neighbors by apartment walls and those white picket fences. What are those fences really for, anyway? It's not the inviting vibe of an open door or a tribal community. On the contrary, it signals mine, my property, keep out, stay over there, stay on your side of the fence.

* * *

Building villages challenges the status quo of modern motherhood which relies on predetermined, one-size-fits-all parameters. Since it is not common to live in an actual village these days, one way that mothers are creating the support that they need is by rejecting the confines of the medical system and seeking alternative systems of care.

I learned that even though I never saw an obstetrician or any doctor until my labor went awry, midwifery in the UK health-care system is not necessarily the same as if I were to find a midwife outside of the system. For example, I never saw the same midwife consistently. I was just seen by whoever happened to be scheduled on the day and the care relationship was built on my file rather than through my personhood.

Robina Khalid received her Masters of Midwifery at SUNY Downstate and founded her homebirth practice, Small Things Grow Midwifery in 2017. She is licensed by the Medical Board of New York State and she is a member of the New York City Homebirth Collective.

In an interview, Khalid helped me better understand the roles of a midwife and doula and why an expectant mother could benefit from the support of both: "Midwives are healthcare professionals. My license is full scope: primacy care, pregnancy, birth, postpartum, and neonatal care. My role as it is traditionally thought of as clinical. A doula is someone that understands birth and supports birth but is not giving clinical care."

These women were the ones throughout history that would attend births. And it was not that long ago that pregnancy became more medicalized and industrialized. According to Khalid: "The change is very much linked to our history of enslavement and immigration, because OBs here went out of their way to stigmatize midwives after the Civil War because Black midwives who were now free were now their competition economically. OBs capitalized on racism because most of the midwives in the country were either Black, Indigenous or from immigrant communities that were not yet considered white. It was essentially a capitalization of racism, as well as eugenics and abortion because midwives traditionally had performed abortion services in an unstigmatized way. So white OBs preyed upon the fear of racist Anglo Saxons in the United States that with emancipation, white people were going to lose their power because more Black people were going to have kids and takeover. And so there was an investment in taking away abortion services."

The advent of modern obstetrics buoyed by racism, a topic we first introduced in Chapter 2, replaced what once was the woman-led, woman-centered practice of birth. We can see the roots of the medical racism faced by Black expectant mothers as well as the beginnings of where we find ourselves today, post the overturning of *Roe vs. Wade* during a time when women's reproductive rights have been reduced to political ammunition.

As well, we must consider the motives of our health-care system generally, a system which Khalid refers to as the Medical Industrial Complex. This term contextualizes the reality that our health and well-being in this country are contingent on someone else making a profit. Can medicine really be about our health when it's tied to money? The National Library of Medicine reports that "in the 1980s the editor of The New England Journal of Medicine coined the term 'medical-industrial complex' to indicate the growing and equally worrying association between doctors and industrial sectors, especially the pharmaceutical industry."[10] It only takes watching one segment of commercials on American TV to see how much money is poured into pushing prescription drugs. Sometimes I can't help but shout at the TV, "Why am I being sold prescription medicine like I'm choosing a laundry detergent?"

Add to this the concerning statistic provided by the American Hospital Association in 2025 that of a total of 6,093 hospitals in the United States, nearly 20 percent (1,214) are for profit.[11] Healthcare is a universal human right, but what happens when it's put into a corporatized, capitalized framework? There is an obvious and inherently problematic conflict of interest between a person's health and the hospital's bottom line.

Khalid explains, "Part of why the United States has evolved in this way is because of our insurance system. We are a for-profit system as opposed to some places like the UK which has nationalized healthcare, which means that they are invested in birth costing less money, having less interventions. In the US, in a private model, there's no reason to invest in stuff like that, which is why we have so many interventions in our births. And the things that actually improved infant and maternal mortality was not anything related to obstetrics, but mostly related to larger medical advancements like antibiotics and better antihemorrhagics. And also really importantly, the ability to screen and treat hypertensive disorders in pregnancy. Obstetrics has really rolled with this idea that if not for us, all the moms and babies would die. And the thing about obstetrics is it has decided that the floor is the goal, which is an alive baby. They say healthy baby, but they actually don't mean healthy baby. They mean an alive baby. And obviously that's everyone's most important goal but when we look at risk, obstetrics is looking at the ultimate risk being a dead baby, as in, that is the only risk that matters. And we're not looking at any of the long-term sequelae that happen from birth in which harm or abuse has been enacted. What we should be focusing on is what is the long-term health of this birth giver and baby?"

If the goal of childbirth is solely an alive baby, it makes sense that there would be little concern for all that happens aside from having an alive baby. We are then not considering the mental or physical health of the mother. No wonder I kept getting the memo to just be grateful that I had a baby. There was no capacity for the related grief, fear, or trauma.

I also felt an undeniable disconnect between how my medical care saw and valued me while I was pregnant versus after I had the baby. When you're pregnant, you are given a schedule of appointments, with all kinds of tests, guidance, and support. If you're considered to be of advanced maternal age like I was for my second pregnancy, you're given even more support, more sonograms, more assurance that you are being cared for. The message is that you as a pregnant person are important.

After the baby is born, all of that support all but vanishes. There is no continuity from the before times through to the after times. The focus from within the health-care system now fully shifts to the baby, and while this makes sense because babies are vulnerable and completely reliant on their caregivers to keep them alive, it would ultimately benefit everyone if there was a more holistic and inclusive perspective of care. Otherwise the painful message to the mother is that she is irrelevant now, reduced to having been a vessel for childbirth.

A midwife like Khalid or a doula like Simpo bridge these breaks in care. Their work shows us a model of how birth used to be—for starters, there is an understanding that it's not just about the literal birth of the baby. There is another equally significant birth—the birth of a mother.

But what if hiring a doula or a midwife is not accessible? Are there other ways that mothers can find and create this kind of care, community, and village?

I believe it starts from understanding and acknowledging that the current way is not working. We need to identify what is missing and broken so that we can start to find solutions.

Our modern life is such that most extended families are not only not living in multigenerational homes, we are often not even living in the same state. Our hyperindividualistic pursuits tend to lead us down our own sequestered paths and into our own nuclear families. Who is the model of the nuclear family ultimately serving? Why is the nuclear family pushed onto us? What is it that is actually being produced and sold?

Khalid points to the time period of 1900–1920 to answer this question, making connections between the nuclear family, the Industrial Revolution, and the period when modern obstetrics took over: "The baby is the product of obstetrics. The baby is a future laborer within capitalism. If you look at the evolution of the nuclear family, it starts being propagandized and pushed right around the time of the Industrial Revolution, because individual households are less efficient and better for capitalism. They consume more than an extended network.

"The nuclear family also isolates people from each other. We end up thinking that all of the challenges we're facing are individual to us. We think the experiences that we struggle with are individual to us and we must be doing something wrong if something is hard. Whereas if you're living in a village or in an extended household, you're seeing different people move through different life stages at different times. And it's normalized that certain moments are hard, certain moments are easy."

It is within the village that we can center the well-being of mothers. It is within the village that we can make space for the gratitude of an alive baby as well as for the validation of grief. It is where we can live in a way that rejects racism, sexism, capitalism, and loneliness.

We need to connect more to each other. We need to look beyond standardized offerings of care, which are boundaried by insurance and profitability. We must interrogate what society tells us we should be doing, including the myth of the mother that does it all, and all by herself.

What if we considered that asking for help doesn't make us weak but rather means we are curious about connection? I know for me, when someone reaches out to me for help, it gives me a sense of joy and purpose to be able to do something for someone else. Never have I thought less of the person asking for help. Instead, what I feel from them is a trust in me, in my humanity. What is created in this exchange is a connection, a bond, a relationship.

This is what we are built for.

These days, I envision creating an actual commune somewhere on this magnificent planet. I've been planting seeds of manifestation: Let's all move to the rural countryside and be farmers! Where the children and animals can roam freely and safely! Where we all take care of each other outside of transactional expectations!

I don't know how realistic of a dream this is, but in the meantime, I know that we were never meant to mother in a singular family unit. The more I have come to understand this, the less stress and overwhelm I have felt in my role as a mother. We need each other. We have always needed each other.

6

Influenced

"Do you plan on breastfeeding?" a midwife asks me at a prenatal checkup.

"Oh, yes, of course!" I gush, as if there could possibly be any other answer. I had absorbed the image of what an ideal mother looked like and I knew it started with effortlessly, happily, and *exclusively* breastfeeding my baby on demand.

"How long will you breastfeed for?"

"At least one year," I answer. It would surely be as easy as simply setting a schedule.

When I was pregnant, I believed the posters all over the doctor's office that read "breast is best" and warned of nipple confusion with images of bottle teats and pacifiers crossed out with the universally understood NO symbol. The mom content I consumed on social media echoed this pressure to #EBF (exclusively breastfeed) if you wanted to be the most perfect, most "natural" mother. #EBF moms posted photos of themselves nursing their babies, as if they were always having the most blissful experience. Rarely did anyone share about the maddening exhaustion, frustration, and physical pain that often comes with trying to breastfeed.

NICU Nurse Sarah Chung revealed a darker side that can accompany this push for mothers to breastfeed: "Certain hospitals want to become magnet. And to become magnet, you have to be breastfeeding friendly. So they want you to breastfeed your baby. But it can be so stressful. Everybody assumes breastfeeding is so easy, but not for a mom that has a premature baby and can't produce milk. And another thing is that it comes down to money because formula costs a lot of money. So it saves the hospital money to push breastfeeding rather than to stock formula. It's so terrible."

It had never occurred to me that the emphasis on breastfeeding could be about anything other than out of best interest for mothers and their babies. It also hadn't occurred to me that what's best for the baby might not be the best for the mother. It just seemed obvious—since it was the most *natural* option—that exclusively breastfeeding was what I would do.

Never mind that I didn't know how to set myself up for successful breastfeeding, like making sure I was drinking copious amounts of water and eating enough so that my body had a better chance at producing milk. What I saw on social media made it seem so easy, so natural; I assumed my body would just make it happen. I was more fixated on what I had always heard about breastfeeding contributing to weight loss, and with my obsessive tendencies around food, I figured breastfeeding and dieting would be a fast track to getting my pre-baby body back.

I didn't understand that sometimes it is not enough to simply *want* to breastfeed your baby.

I'd seen my yoga mentor wear her newborn in a sling and nurse him—*while* she was teaching class. I'd heard stories from my friends who had to buy an extra freezer to store all the extra milk they were pumping. I held a lot of assumptions in my mind but in reality, I knew nothing. I didn't know that milk didn't necessarily come in right away.

I didn't know that babies don't always instinctively latch. I didn't know that I would be squeezing drops of breastmilk into a syringe to feed my baby.

Although I had been okay with midwives giving him bottles of formula while we were in the hospital, I refused to give him formula once we were discharged. He was unsettled and didn't sleep well. At his one month checkup, we learned that he had lost too much weight. My attachment to exclusively breastfeeding was actually causing harm to my baby.

We immediately started mix-feeding him after that checkup, but with every bottle I made and fed him, I felt like a failure. I wished so badly that I could be like so many other moms who seemed to breastfeed with such ease. And if a mother can't properly—exclusively—breastfeed her baby, then, what good of a mother is she?

*   *   *

I had no idea what I was doing from the moment I knew I was pregnant. My own mother was never going to be someone I could turn to. So I found myself following moms on social media—*momfluencers*—that I could learn from and aspire to emulate.

I couldn't have made a worse decision for my mental health.

This was 2014, and the savviness we social media users have now (or at least some of us) was a long way off.

Instead of feeling inspired, I felt awful. My home, hair, body—even my baby—looked nothing like what I was seeing.

There's one particular image I don't think I'll ever forget: a mother and baby, probably about eight months old, in a meticulously designed kitchen. The mother in a beautiful dress, looking like she had just been to Drybar for a blowout. The baby was smiling, sitting on the kitchen island. The mother was not in arm's length of the baby, and she looked unconcerned about her child, who could roll off the counter at any moment.

In my raw, vulnerable, anxious state, I believed what I saw. Why couldn't I create this scene, have that hair, fit into a nice, non-maternity dress, be carefree and happy? What was wrong with me that my life looked nothing like this? Everywhere I looked, my brain was repeatedly getting the message that I was not good enough, I did not look right, I was not mothering right.

I couldn't stop looking.

In those early months, I didn't recognize myself at all. My postpartum body didn't have the cuteness that my pregnant body had. I wasn't used to not having the freedom to shower when I wanted to. My hormones wreaked havoc. I couldn't keep up with household chores. Simply leaving the house felt overwhelming. I felt isolated. My phone became an extension of myself more than it ever had been—a lifeline to the outside world.

This season of early motherhood is a vulnerable time for most new mothers—it certainly was for me. No matter how many books I may have read while pregnant, how many babies were already in my life as nieces, nephews, or godchildren, or how innately nurturing I considered myself, there was just no preparing for how I would feel as a mother to *my* new baby.

Although I didn't know it at the time, I wasn't alone in feeling lost and unsupported during this time. The American College of Obstetricians and Gynecologists (ACOG) states, "The weeks following birth are a critical period for a woman and her infant, setting the stage for long-term health and well-being. During this period, a woman is adapting to multiple physical, social, and psychological changes . . . this 'fourth trimester' can present considerable challenges for women, including lack of sleep, fatigue, pain, breastfeeding difficulties, stress, new onset or exacerbation of mental health disorders, lack of sexual desire, and urinary incontinence."[1]

As such, the ACOG emphasizes the importance of postpartum checkups because "many moms struggle with anxiety, pain, fatigue, and other concerns."[2] I was offered one paltry postpartum checkup and while they now advise that "new moms connect with their ob-gyns several times during the 12 weeks after birth," up to 40 percent of new mothers do not even attend one postpartum visit. Of those that do, less than 50 percent "reported that they received enough information at the visit about postpartum depression, birth spacing, healthy eating, the importance of exercise, or changes in their sexual response and emotions."[3]

A 2023 postpartum survey by BabyCenter and economist and parenting expert Emily Oster reported on the ways new moms are overlooked and impacted by a lack of social and systemic support. Only 41 percent of mothers feel they have enough support during the postpartum period, and anyway, that support centers around caring for their newborn—not themselves. Moms of color are disproportionately more likely to feel unsupported: 22 percent of AAPI mothers and 32 percent of Black mothers feel they have the support they need compared to 44 percent of white mothers.[4]

And despite the ubiquitous saying, "It takes a village!"—how many of us actually have the privilege of a village? For immigrant families, there is often an internal diaspora within individual families, especially if there has been a break in the family unit due to generational trauma or due to children moving away from their parents in order to find better education or job opportunities. Even if said sacred village is available, our culture preaches the importance of the independent woman, the woman who has and does it all.

I personally rejected the idea of help in any form. I feared being criticized, shamed, or looked down upon to the point where it was not even an option for me to feel overwhelmed as a new mother. American values have always rewarded individual achievements and toxic positivity—that can-do attitude. I would impress everyone with how good—how naturally, effortlessly, inherently good—I would be at mothering. I had taken care of myself up until this point and I was wiser and more mature now. It seemed logical to think that I wouldn't need support.

Yet in that so-called fourth trimester, I had a cascade of questions without easy answers. What does my baby need? How much milk should I be feeding him? Is he sleeping enough? Does that cry mean that he's too hot or that he needs a cuddle? The idea of a "mother's instinct" felt oppressive—a suggestion that I should innately know what my baby needed at all times. Where would I turn to for support, for community?

As I navigated this new world, life around me didn't stop. The framework of life itself—with its twenty-four-hour days, the need for the parents to at the very least themselves eat, sleep, and go to the bathroom, and money being necessary for survival—had not changed. Stuck in the tyranny of meeting an entirely new set of needs without enough hours in the day, I was learning it all on the job. I couldn't pause my baby while honing my skills of making a bottle at just the right temperature, becoming proficient with the breast pump, or employing the five S's of the "happiest baby on the block." There was no break, no release of tension, no end.

I was plagued with uncertainty about every little thing I did. I was never sure if the bath water was too hot or too cold. I was so neurotic about mixing formula correctly that I would lose count of scoops midway through and have to start over, throwing away the formula I had already scooped out. I could not for the life of me interpret one type of cry from another; it all grated my very soul. And I found myself without reliable guidance: There was completely contradictory advice from all angles. I didn't have the confidence or experience within myself, so I naturally looked to outside resources—books, experts, friends—and was often left more perplexed.

Instagram had been introduced four years before my son was born. We were accustomed to unsolicited vacation albums commandeering our feeds but we weren't yet savvy enough to understand that those Insta-squares were showing but a tiny part of someone's life. As a new mom looking for advice, inspiration, and community, I unwittingly followed mommy bloggers and what we now call momfluencers. I reasoned that if someone had tens of thousands of followers, they must be important—experts even. The images of motherhood they were portraying looked fun, beautiful, and perfect. They seemed to have the answers.

The comparisons and feelings of inadequacy started immediately. Why don't I look as good as that mom? Why doesn't my baby look as happy as that baby? Why is my home a mess?

Those picture-perfect posts are the ones that typically garner lots of likes and positive comments, so the social proof is clear: These moms are succeeding. You put pressure on yourself to do more. And as I saw so many times over, the comparison turns to competition: *I* had a "natural" birth, *I* exclusively breastfeed, *we* co-sleep, *we* do baby-led weaning. (These competitions don't ever seem to stop: Mothers of older children were just as likely to partake. *My* kid does sixteen after-school activities, *my* kid is trilingual, *my* kid got into an Ivy League.)

I didn't understand then that bombarding myself with all this manufactured narrative about motherhood was impacting my mental health. (The impact of social media on mothers is well-documented, and can lead to comparison, despair, feelings of inadequacy, and more.[5]) I was too tired to apply any critical thinking to what I was seeing—of course she's used photoshop, of course she isn't doing it all alone, of course she has moments of struggle too. Instead, I blindly wanted to be like the images I saw, even if it was pulling me underwater and I was running out of air.

*   *   *

The women I followed represented expertise: They had the answers I needed. And I could become the kind of mother they were if I simply followed—and bought—their examples.

If I'm a mom feeling tired and overwhelmed, I might follow a mom who seems to have it all figured out. Get my hair blown out weekly, get all those makeup products for that no-makeup-makeup look, and get seventy-five baskets for storing toys which of course must only be made of natural material and in neutral colors, and that designer diaper bag, and definitely that peasant dress, and the Cartier Love bangle—the list goes on.

If I'm a mom feeling unseen and invalidated, I might follow proud stay-at-home moms or "tradmoms" who glorify housework like laundry, cooking, and cleaning. If I can just build out a laundry room/ mudroom combo and buy that cooking appliance(s) and how about that $600 vacuum, I could be like them.

If I'm a working mom feeling guilty about not spending enough time with my children, I might follow the career mom who shares solutions to being in two places at once. Ask to work from home for half the time. Create a daycare program within your office. Bring your baby to meetings, and accuse people of bigotry if they have a problem with your need to breastfeed in boardrooms. Do it all, and if you don't, you've failed as a mother. (This rings of the many ways even in modern history that mothers are demonized for their inadequacies. See: blaming a child's autism on their mother's supposed coldness.[6])

Want the perfect birth? A birth team includes privately procured midwives and birth doulas. Maybe a placenta encapsulist (though, there are no money back guarantees if your placenta ends up tainted like mine did). A maternity night nurse and a private lactation consultant who makes house calls. Postpartum massage, craniosacral adjustments, pelvic floor healing—none of which is covered by insurance, of course. A personal trainer and private chef, or at least a Sakara subscription. Most mothers cannot afford any of this, but we are being inundated with images that suggest that we should be able to. We just need to follow, lean in, work harder, manifest, consume, and repeat. Momfluencers pull us into the endless, impossible, destructive cycle of capitalism.

We're left thinking: *Maybe with the perfect products, I can be the perfect mother.*

* * *

In the year my son was born, I had an entirely different view of race than I do now. I believed Asian Americans like me were as American as anyone else; people just didn't see color, right? Adhering to the model minority myth fell neatly in with our cultural tendency of saving face, of brushing any issues under the rug, of not talking about hard things.

Trayvon Martin had been murdered at age seventeen, two years prior, and a shift was on the horizon but had yet to materialize for me. There was, for the first time, a growing understanding that mothers of color, especially Black mothers, experience parenting differently than white mothers. Still, white mothers ruled the conversation.

As I scrolled social media, searching for connection, it didn't even occur to me that most of the mothers showing up in my feeds were white. Without realizing it, I was being served a constant reminder that I was not like those women.

I think about what that image I saw on Instagram—with the perfect mother, perfect kitchen, perfect baby perched on the counter—wanted me to believe. It showed a world without danger, where nothing could ever happen to you or your baby. It showed a world that doesn't exist for anyone who isn't white—or financially privileged—in this country.

As an Asian American with immigrant parents, I have always been aware that I was part of the minority. Daily life reminded me of this, from looking different to most of my classmates, to seeing my parents being treated differently, and to all the white-centric media that was inherently part of my childhood. In the few places that Asians were portrayed on TV, we were always shown as weird, nerdy, uncool—as outsiders.

As I dug deeper into my social media obsession, one image kept appearing: white, cisgender, heterosexual, Christian, slender, able-bodied, financially stable, educated, and not an immigrant. It was a constant reminder of what I was not and what I could never be. I didn't understand white supremacy like I do today, and I assumed the oppression or rejection I felt had to do with my own personal failings as a mother.

*   *   *

It was a conversation with a close friend of mine that helped me understand this intersection of race, identity, and motherhood. She is a white mother who had a very close and loving relationship with her mother. Her own daughter is blonde and blue-eyed, characteristics I've always commented on, almost unconsciously figuring that her daughter's life will be so much easier than my children's lives. "She's so lucky," I would think. "She won't get teased for having slanted eyes or dark skin. She won't stick out like a sore thumb in class photos. She'll probably be popular and people will think she's beautiful. She'll get into colleges more easily, get job opportunities more easily. There will always be more space for her than for my children."

I shared with my friend an early version of this chapter about momfluencers. She responded, "It feels worth mentioning your postpartum depression. Without the caveat of the postpartum mental health piece, I find myself pushing against the narrative."

I was struck by her response. She thinks it's only people with postpartum mental illness that are negatively affected by social media?

I was sure we were simply having a misunderstanding. Had she missed all the headlines about the detrimental effects of social media? Had she really never felt bad about herself after seeing perfect mom posts? Maybe she was an exception; what about her friends?

She cited three of her close mom friends who, like her, were never bothered by what they saw on social media, at least not when it came to motherhood. And that's when it hit me: all of these moms are white and financially secure.

This isn't to say that white moms aren't also impacted by toxic momfluencer culture, which inherently excludes anyone without discretionary income, like the 60 percent of Americans living paycheck to paycheck.[7] But what I have come to understand more clearly is part of why the social media motherhood landscape is so treacherous for me: After a lifetime of constantly being told that I did not belong and that I wasn't good enough, the barrage of visual reminders through Instagram when what I most needed was support and encouragement as a new mother was too much.

I innately, if not explicitly, understood that I could never be like these momfluencers. But instead of understanding that from a critical thinking lens that takes into account systems of oppression, I internalized it all. It became ammunition for my self-hate, always available, like an anvil pulling me deeper into postpartum depression.

What the influencer economy—including the companies paying them—know and count on is that we care about our children and we want to do everything we can to give them the best life possible. They prey on this as much as they do on our vulnerability and naivete, fueled by patriarchal expectations of perfection, especially if we're a first-time mom.

I don't want to see these momfluencers—the ones who make clear that I cannot be the perfect mother—but it's in social media platforms' interest to keep showing them to me. Jessica Grose writes in the *New York Times* that "momfluencers, the purveyors of these pernicious expectations, are part of a multibillion-dollar industry, selling products to a market of millennial moms with an estimated $2 trillion to spend."[8] When you can shop through the in-app stores on Instagram or TikTok, they profit.

I could spend all the money I have trying to buy their lives. But I will never be white, I will never come from a long line of established Americans. And how about mothers that cannot afford the lifestyle sold by momfluencers? We will never know the safety and lack of worry that these mothers show with their babies. By those standards, we will never, ever get it right.

* * *

Several years after Ryker's birth, I saw a popular momfluencer posing for photos in my own neighborhood in New York City—wearing wooly sweaters in the middle of July. It was clearly staged. I kept an eye on this mom's profile, and those photos showed up months later during the fall with a caption suggesting that they had been taken casually that morning.

As much as I may have known that what I was seeing on social media was never the whole story, seeing the fabrication play out so blatantly was jarring, even frightening. What was I buying into? What was I allowing myself to be influenced by?

This moment of truth gave me the kick I needed to finally force myself to look away. And I needed to go cold turkey.

I deleted Instagram and I stayed off of it for two years. When I felt ready to tiptoe back into the digital minefield, I was determined to do so with my eyes wide open, on *my* terms. I cut down the number of accounts I was following to 100. Any posts that made me feel badly about myself, I immediately unfollowed.

I started following moms who were unabashedly sharing unfiltered photos of their "imperfect" postpartum bodies, messy homes, and other real aspects of motherhood. These moms made me feel less alone, and they gave me strength to feel like I could take on challenges. It felt like a community, and even now, I especially love the funny, sarcastic moms who say out loud the stuff most of us think but feel like we cannot say. I found a new take on breastfeeding—"*fed* is best"—that would have changed everything for me in those early days when I was desperate to live up to an impossible model.

Here's what I've realized since: I am not the outlier for feeling this way, whether because I had postpartum depression or because I am not white or because I don't have a trust fund. The outliers are those social media moms that are perpetuating lies—or at the very least, deeply skewed realities—at the expense of the rest of us, regardless of how we identify. We are all impacted, whether we are aware of it or not.

And that momfluencer in the wooly sweater at the height of a New York City summer? Years after I saw her posing for that post, she has since deleted her digital footprint and declared bankruptcy. What truth had all the glitz and glamour been hiding?

Many mothers feel burnout, whether they consider themselves a stay-at-home mom or a working mom. Moms are overwhelmed by the expectation that they do it all, be it all, provide it all, while looking and acting like they haven't gone through the single most transformative experience of their lives. Moms are enraged by the capitalistic patriarchy that holds them to impossible standards while reducing systemic infrastructure of childcare. Inflation is higher than it's ever been while women continue to be paid less than men. Moms are rightfully angry.

When we express our anger, we're criticized for being irrational, unstable. If we repress our anger, it will inevitably insist on expressing itself through physical maladies or emotional distress or both. And then we are blamed, systemically scapegoated to divert attention away from the real issues of institutional lack and oppression.

This paradigm affects all mothers, even those who see themselves more closely reflected in online narratives or blockbuster films, because nobody is perfect. Nobody's real life looks like the perfectly curated profiles the algorithm so innocently invites us to explore. This hurts white mothers, BIPOC mothers, mothers of all socioeconomic statuses and non-binary birthing people, albeit in different ways, and until we dismantle the perfect mother narrative in all its racist, patriarchal, ableist, capitalistic power, none of us are free.

I wonder what those early months and years would have been like without a constant stream of inadequacy being fed to me. Without my very identity constantly called into question, would I have sunk so deep into depression and anxiety? But it's a catch-22: If I hadn't been grappling with postpartum depression and other mental health challenges, would I have been able to look at those images with a critical eye and not see myself as a failure when I was not reflected in them?

I don't know the answers to those questions, but I'm certain of one thing: Without a visible culture of motherhood that doesn't aspire to whiteness, wealth, thinness, or any other domination, there's more room for all of us to do our best to love our children and ourselves as the mothers we are. In valuing and protecting other types of motherhood—immigrant mothers like mine, poor mothers, Asian or Black or Brown mothers, there is liberation for us all.

7

Heard

I started writing this book several years ago, while I was still experiencing acute symptoms of postpartum depression. I didn't know if I would ever find my way out. I was always in a hyper-vigilant state, worrying about when the next panic attack would hit me. The worry alone would trigger anxiety which would then trigger the panic attack I had been worrying about in the first place.

Therapy was a necessary part of my healing process.

Because there was no medical infrastructure to support maternal mental health through my prenatal and postpartum doctors' appointments, it was a struggle to find therapy in the first place. Almost all pregnant women are screened for gestational diabetes through medically supported, reliable testing. Postpartum mental disorders are more common than gestational diabetes—the CDC reports 8 percent of women who had live births had gestational diabetes compared to its report that 13 percent of *surveyed* women reported depressive symptoms[1]—yet screening for postpartum depression is haphazard at best, if available at all.

Even for those without a postpartum mood disorder diagnosis, the newborn period is overwhelming and isolating for most parents, particularly with your first child. Not everyone has a readymade village; not everyone can afford paid help. You're in the trenches. You can't remember the last time you showered. You can't finish a thought, sentence, or task. And you're downright exhausted.

Mental health support for a new mother is a medical necessity, just as much as your baby's weekly and monthly well visits.

When I found myself drowning and wondering if I was experiencing postpartum depression, I tried to talk to friends and fellow mothers. They would say things like:

"Having children cured me of my depression!"

"This is just how life is with children, you'll get used to it."

"Maybe you need to do more yoga? Meditation? Acupuncture? Sex helps too."

I only felt worse.

I felt like I had ruined my life by having a child and that I was destined to ruin my child's life as well. I figured I didn't deserve to be happy. I was doomed to lose myself to mental illness as my mother had. It was written in my genetic blueprint.

Or maybe it was just baby blues. I didn't know how to discern whether it was just getting accustomed to my new life or something else.

I spoke to LCSW, therapist, educator, and mother Alisha Bennett about this unsettling period after having a baby: "What I think would have been more helpful for me to know before I had a baby is understanding that your body is literally recovering from the most traumatic thing it can go through. Childbirth is trauma. There is a baby going underneath your pelvic bone and out, that is pure fucking physical trauma. Your body is going to be broken, your hormones are at the highest level they can ever be, and think about the moment that you have felt the most tired—you are going to feel that way every single day for months. That's what I wish I had been told but at the same time, I will also say that no one can say anything that's going to really truly prepare you for what it is. So let's at least stop glorifying how beautiful and amazing it is to bring your baby home from the hospital."

What we say to each other matters. It is such a disservice that most of us don't tell each other the truth about what to expect. I find myself still hesitating sometimes, because I don't want to be that negative person. And I'm not sure if it's a lack of empathy or being dissociated from one's own suffering, but we need to get better at listening to and holding space for each other's pain. From health-care workers to friends and partners to society at large, there is so much more we can be doing to care for postpartum mothers.

It can feel like we are all just navigating the minefield of motherhood in the dark.

Psychiatrist Pyarvin Abbasova, who is originally from Russia, couldn't easily identify her own postpartum depression despite the fact that she is a mental health professional: "In Russia, the maternity leave is a year and a half and it starts when you are seven and a half months pregnant. You will not see a single woman in the workplace, unless, maybe you own your own business. Otherwise, those last months of your pregnancy, you're at home, you're getting ready for a baby. Then you are paid 80% of your salary. You even have the option to stay at home for up to three years and your job is held for you.

"When I had my first child, I had an urgent C-section and I went to back to work six weeks later. Everyone I know in Russia was shocked, and I think I was shocked, too. But I had no choice. I had to work because I was the main income provider of the family. My ex-husband was also working so we swapped shifts between work and being home with the baby. This meant I never had a break. I was either working or taking care of the baby.

"Even though I'm a psychiatrist, it was difficult to recognize I had postpartum depression because I honestly just thought that I was so tired and sleep deprived. I could not tell the difference. Am I tired or am I depressed? I feel like I never had the chance to restart because six weeks after an urgent C-section is not enough."

Dr. Abbasova was not prepared to recognize her own postpartum depression because she came from a culture that was designed to give new mothers space to rest without financial burden or worrying about job loss. She figured that she was just exhausted because she had to go back to work so early. Even as a psychiatrist herself, she was unable to see the serious and detrimental effect of not having the time to recover after childbirth and in particular, after an emergency cesarian.

It enables me to have some grace for myself that even a psychiatrist struggled to get mental health help when she needed it the most.

*   *   *

I did try to get help a few months into my motherhood. In the United Kingdom, everything is done through your local GP office, what we call our Primary Care Provider here in the United States. If you need a therapist, you first talk to your GP—who is not someone who necessarily knows you well but rather whoever happens to be in rotation at the time. The tradeoff with benefiting from socialized healthcare is that it is not personalized. I don't think any health care worker knew me by name nor I by theirs. The GP will refer you to the mental health department. You then wait to receive a phone call to determine the severity and urgency of your particular situation.

When my phone call came, my palms went clammy and I could feel my heart pounding in my chest. I knew I had requested—needed, desperately—the help. But I suddenly had a sense of deep distrust. The first questions I was asked were:

Are you having thoughts of self-harm?

Are you having thoughts of harming your baby?

I can't even recall what questions followed because I was so jarred by the way the call had started—the way you might automatically feel guilty in the presence of the police, despite having done nothing wrong.

I answered, "No, of course not!" which was the truth, but I also went on to instinctively downplay the rest of my answers to the questions about how I felt. I was terrified that someone was going to show up at my door and take my baby away from me or take me away from my baby.

The purpose of the call was to triage me and as a result of my watered-down answers, I wasn't given a therapy appointment for another several weeks. The wait time alone gaslit me into thinking that I was fine, or that I at least *should* be fine, otherwise surely there would have been more immediacy in offering me support.

I was still trusting that the system was working and that it would take care of me.

By the time I showed up at my first—and only—therapy appointment in London, I was already extremely disconnected from myself. Filling in the form that asked me to rate feelings of depression felt impossible—how could I assign a number between one and five to something that felt so unquantifiable?

I had become so versed at masking and I was so inexperienced with therapy that I ended up treating the session like a job interview, as if the purpose was to make a good first impression. When the therapist concluded, "It sounds like you just had some baby blues and you've now come out of the haze! You're doing great!"—I lapped it up. Of course I did—I desperately wanted to be okay, to be told I was okay, to be sure that everything would be okay.

At the same time, I left the office feeling uneasy and untethered.

* * *

Mental health was not something discussed in my family, despite my mother's many crises and suicide attempts. To this day, we have only ever had one direct conversation about her mental health, while she lay in a hospital bed in a coma after yet another failed suicide attempt. Other than the family counseling sessions I had insisted on back when I had "run away" from home, where we did not dare discuss my mother's—or anyone's—mental state, therapy was not on the table. It might as well have not existed. Skepticism of therapy is cultural, to be sure—it's not a part of most Asian families' experiences.

In a particularly apt moment on Mindy Kaling's "Never Have I Ever," a Black therapist says to an Indian mom, "I didn't think you were someone who believed in therapy." The Indian mom replies, "I don't. It's for white people."

Therapist, author, and advice columnist for *The Washington Post* Sahaj Kaur Kohli expounds on this cultural disparity in our interview: "It's really important to understand that many of us who train as clinicians in the West are being taught from a Western framework. I really enjoyed my graduate program but I also despised it in a lot of ways as a lot of the tools and techniques and skills we were learning were rooted in Eurocentric values and norms like focusing on individualism when it comes to the client. That's not to say that it's bad, it just leaves out parts of so many of our identities that incorporate collectivism, community, and ancestral healing—all of these things that we are not taught in those professional graduate programs. And so a lot of that I had to learn myself as a daughter of Indian immigrants, a daughter of refugees. I've learned from my own family about the stigma of mental health, whether it's because my own parents struggle to talk about their feelings or from hearing stories about relatives who have passed away who might have had mental health struggles. And I think that stigma is passed down. It's so inherent and so internalized for so many of us, even if you are unlearning it and you believe in mental health care. A lot of us are struggling with these narratives that mental health care is a sign of failure. It's a sign of weakness. It can bring shame to your family. And you also have the systemic stereotypes that reinforce the stigma, like the model minority myth that as Asian Americans we are seen as successful, productive, submissive, agreeable. All of these things that we can end up internalizing as Asian Americans."

Beyond the personal and familial barriers of mental health illiteracy and unfamiliarity, even if therapy had been something my family wanted to pursue, it's unlikely that we would have been able to find what we needed. My father would have been navigating a foreign country's approach to mental health—one that is specifically *not* designed for us. This experience is all too common: An alarming number of people who may wish to seek therapy simply can't. There's a dual-faceted inaccessibility: Logistics—like cost or language barriers—*and* a lack of cultural competency. It's clear that our mental health is interwoven with our identities, and when therapists are unaware of those nuances, the care can be inadequate. (An American Psychological Association Report reveals that a staggering 86 percent of therapists are white.[2])

Not only that: Asking for help in a therapeutic setting can lead to unjust criminalization, especially for BIPOC mothers. There are so many people who need help and so few places to safely get it.

All things considered, I have been one of the lucky ones in being able to benefit from therapy to address my upbringing and postpartum mental health. Being born in the West, fluent in English, and financially relatively secure, I have had the privilege to access care—however imperfect it may have been—as I navigate years of trauma and motherhood.

*   *   *

It would be more than a year before I sought mental health support again. By then, we had moved to New York City and I had been a mother for eighteen months. What I was feeling could no longer be categorized as baby blues, I was sure of that much.

The panic attacks were so terrifying and suffocating that I could no longer repress, deny, or pretend. I couldn't sit still during a routine dental cleaning. I cried to my acupuncturist when she left me alone to *relax* in the treatment room, shouting out that I was scared. My nervous system wouldn't allow me to sleep so I often ended up pacing or cleaning the apartment in the middle of the night.

Finally, I told my husband, "I think I need help."

I called around to a few therapists and I made an appointment to see the first one who happened to return my call. My only criteria was immediacy. I ended up seeing him for nearly eight years. There was something about his stoic, somewhat stern demeanor that was beneficial to me: I think it was in some ways culturally familiar, a digression from the "I see your heart" or "holding space" language that dominates therapy and speaks primarily to whiteness.

As the weeks passed, it was intrinsically grounding to learn that I just had to survive and manage symptoms from one session to the next. I might have a panic attack on a Friday but if I could just hold on for a few days until my next session on Wednesday, I would be okay.

It's the thought of the endlessness and aloneness of suffering that feels unbearable.

I was never suicidal. I'm not sure if the reason is because I had witnessed my mom attempt to take her life so many times and I had experienced the ripple effect of terror that caused us as family. I could never do that to my children and to my husband. But living through panic attacks and under the oppressive fear of panic attacks felt truly torturous.

I thought about the absurdity of the phrase "life's too short." Too short? No, a life of suffering feels too long.

*   *   *

Therapy helped me dissect and understand my psyche—past and present—and how I might be able to shape my future state of mind. I learned to separate myself as the thinker of thoughts and the feeler of feelings rather than as the thoughts and the feelings themselves. I learned about the timelessness of trauma—that the brain does not always recognize that the traumatic thing is not happening right now, and so it sends off warning signals by way of fight, flight, or freeze. I learned to start trusting myself as the narrator of my own life.

None of this is easy. Especially because we exist in relationships not only with ourselves but with our partners, families, and communities. We all have to navigate our collective reality, which is a living, changing thing. Mothers, especially, are constantly multitasking, compartmentalizing, and learning on the job.

The work may start on your therapist's couch, but you must continue it in your own way. It helped me to think about nurturing my mental health the same way I try to show up for my friends: over a cup of coffee, offering my thoughtful attention with love, reserving judgment and criticism.

Each week was an excavation. I had started by asking for help accepting the traumatic birth of my son, thinking that was the root cause of my suffering. I was genuinely shocked when I learned it went way further back than that, back to my childhood.

I had no idea that all this time, I had been relying on coping mechanisms to live with the trauma of my childhood—the trauma of having had a mentally ill mother, compounded by other generational, immigrant, and racial traumas. Therapy was like cleaning out a basement that I didn't even know existed.

What had once felt like karmic punishment—my shredded nervous system and loss of self—turned out to be, at the risk of sounding incredibly cliché, the greatest gift. Postpartum depression ended up being a most potent invitation for me to live in truth. Portraying perfection was no longer my goal. Instead, I became interested in accepting and responding to what actually is. That's where I started finding peace.

In being forced to look at myself and my "stuff," I realized there was so much that I didn't actually know about myself. I think I had been so afraid of what I might discover that I kept a lot hidden. The persona I had crafted felt safe: a successful yoga teacher who accepted her dysfunctional past, who had her life, her body, and her personality under control. I was most definitely a model minority. Who knew what I would find if I allowed that veneer to crack apart?

But it was in breaking down and apart that I learned that I needed to love myself. And I learned that my capacity to love myself is no different to the unconditional love a parent has for their child. I just had never been taught this.

In order to heal, that which is holding us back from healing does need to come up and out, to be processed by our mind *and body*. As the saying goes, we have to feel it to heal it. It's like any physical detoxing process. It will be uncomfortable, even painful. But undoubtedly— better out than in.

None of this means that there is one solution for everyone. There should be as many healing plans as there are people on the planet— one size most definitely does not fit all. In a best-case scenario, you have a supportive family unit—no, a village—medical and psychological care, and the finances to cover everything you need. But this is likely far from reality for most of us. If we are suffering from one or more postpartum mental health issues—which include postpartum anxiety/OCD/panic/PTSD as well as postpartum mental health issues experienced by non-birthing partners, including men—the lack of any one of those supports is probably part of why we find ourselves in postpartum darkness in the first place.

Ultimately, I learned that I needed to advocate for myself. I personally decided against medication, but it is important to state that medication can be an absolutely necessary part of healing. Therapist Alisha Bennett shared in our conversation that for her, therapy alone did not help her postpartum anxiety: "It was beyond therapy. I'm not saying this is true for everyone. I do think people regulate in their own ways based on childhood trauma. But I didn't feel better until I started taking Lexapro when my daughter was three months old. It fucking changed who I was as a mother, who I was as a person. All of the noise was gone. It's like balancing out your brain chemicals and chemistry. Now that I am on the other side of it four years later, I wish I would have started taking Lexapro when I was 25 years old. The amount of time, energy, and mental space that I could have had . . . I could have had a decade of a different state.

"I even had a very good friend who used to work for the Motherhood Center. Someone very well-versed in postpartum and understanding what moms need and everything about mom-related mental health. I would call her and she would give me strategies and nothing helped. Nothing. Nothing could get me from that state, that hyper-vigilant, hyperactive state of anxiety that I was in. Until I took medication."

Bennett found what worked for her. We each have to find what works for us. My decision against medication was rooted in my mother's dependency on and multiple overdoses of medication. For me, medication was deeply triggering and if I'm honest, it continues to be. Therapy, journaling, and sharing my story—this became my way out, when I found the language to understand and the courage to express what I was experiencing. I was also lucky to have an existing somatic and spiritual practice, even though not everything worked all the time.

Communication and connection continue to play an essential role in taking care of my mental health. There can be an almost immediate sense of relief from simply knowing you are not alone.

*   *   *

Babies are being born every single day. It is crucial that there are systems of support for the mental and physical health and well-being for all the mothers being born into their motherhood.

The CDC reported 3,659,289 births in the United States in 2020—an increase of 1 percent from the previous year—and a fertility rate of 56.6 births per 1,000 women ages 15–44.[3] Worldwide, the UN estimates around 385,000 babies are born each day, a number that's expected to remain relatively stable through 2070.[4] In other words, a huge chunk of the global population has recently given birth, with each person experiencing their own unique struggles and challenges rooted in their unique life experiences, with many of these challenges exacerbated or intensified by the pandemic and other dysregulating current events—many of which disproportionately affect BIPOC birthing parents and others who hold marginalized identities.

For example, research by the University of Michigan School of Nursing found that postpartum depression (PPD) rose nearly *three-fold* during the pandemic.[5] According to PostpartumDepression.org, in the United States alone, 10–20 percent of people who have live births will experience PPD, and it is estimated that 50 percent of mothers with PPD are not formally diagnosed by a health professional.[6] The CDC reports 950,000 people per year suffering from PPD, but this only accounts for self-reported cases.[7]

How many people have not acknowledged their PPD out of shame or fear? It's estimated that 1.3 million people per year are likely suffering from some type of postpartum mood disorder. For comparison: 800,000 women are currently living with diabetes (National Diabetes Information Clearinghouse), 300,000 have experienced a stroke (CDC), and 230,000 have been diagnosed with breast cancer (National Cancer Institute).[8]

Where is the infrastructure of support for postpartum mental health?

To put it simply, as the Maternal Mental Health Leadership Alliance states: *maternal mental health conditions are the most common complication of pregnancy and parenting.*[9] Other relevant statistics include:

- In Canada: 23 percent of new mothers experience PPD or postpartum anxiety. For mothers aged twenty-five years and younger, this statistic rises to 30 percent.

- In the UK: 1/10 people who give birth experience PPD, 1/8 experience depression during pregnancy, and 25 percent of these individuals continue to experience symptoms after their baby turns one.

- 50 percent of men whose partners are diagnosed with PPD go on to have depression themselves.

- 50–75 percent of birthing parents report experiencing the "baby blues" 1–2 weeks postpartum.

- 17 percent experience postpartum anxiety within the first three months postpartum and 75 percent of those with PPD also have postpartum anxiety.

- 3–5 percent of birthing parents experience postpartum OCD for at least 6 months after giving birth.

- 7 percent experience postpartum panic disorder, with symptoms occurring anytime within the first year.

- 30 percent of those who had a complication during pregnancy or delivery experience PPD.

- 1–2/1,000 women birthing parents experience postpartum psychosis.[10]

Over the past decade, suicide attempts during/after pregnancy have tripled, and 60 percent of those who died by suicide had not seen a mental health care provider within the month.[11] How many deaths were due to mothers feeling utterly alone?

Despite these sobering statistics, those suffering from postpartum mental health struggles often receive little support. As we saw with Bennett, while medication can be a godsend for some, it doesn't work for everyone, and options (not to mention access) can be limited. According to Scientific American:

Many women who suffer from postpartum depression receive standard antidepressants, including selective serotonin reuptake inhibitors such as Prozac. It is unclear how well these drugs work, however, because the neurotransmitter serotonin may play only a secondary role in the condition or may not be involved at all.[12]

The National Library of Medicine (NLM) reports:

Numerous studies have reported on the low rates of screening, diagnosis, and treatment of perinatal depression in medical settings. Clinician discomfort with psychiatric disorders, time constraints, low belief in maternal mental health having an important effect on child development, and lack of knowledge about resources are some of the barriers to clinician screening for psychiatric disorders in medical settings.[13]

Socioeconomic factors, race, and ethnicity also play a major role in access to care. According to the NLM:

> *9% of white women initiated postpartum mental health care in comparison to 4% of Black women and 5% of Latina women. Black and Latina mothers are also less likely to receive follow-up treatment/continued care. There are [also] significant racial-ethnic differences in depression-related mental health care after delivery. Suboptimal treatment was prevalent among all low-income women; however, racial disparities in the initiation and continuation of PPD care are troubling and warrant clinical and policy attention.* (It's also worth noting that this particular study does not even include other women of color.)[14]

To look at the big picture, only 50 percent[15] of those diagnosed with PPD receive treatment. And as many as 40 percent[16] don't attend a postpartum visit, with the number almost certainly being higher for those with limited resources.

*   *   *

We need better systems of mental health care, period. We need to normalize conversations around mental hygiene. In the same way that we talk about taking care of our physical bodies from what we eat to what kind of exercise we do to mentioning when we've had a doctor's appointment, we need to be talking about our mental state and feelings. What feels like a struggle right now? What feels scary right now? What kind of support could we use right now?

We need to question why society puts so much more emphasis on caring for our bodies than it does caring for our minds and our spirits. Through a practice like yoga—and any other type of movement inviting your conscious attention—you can viscerally experience how the mind and body are connected. They impact each other; in fact, they can never not impact each other. We are made up of both.

So to go through the most physically transformative experience a human body can go through—pregnancy and childbirth—and not receive mental and emotional care is quite simply—illogical.

I think what's particularly hard with mental health care is that there really is no magic pill that works for all, no scientifically proven one right answer for all. Physical health care similarly has inconsistencies, of course; medicine is not an exact science. For example, we understand that certain people have allergic reactions to medications that the majority of people are fine with. But with physical health care it tends to be a case of exceptions and not the rule—if you're the one with the allergic reaction, you're likely the outlier.

It's different with mental health care because our mental state comes down to our uniqueness as individuals, so there is no "rule." Mental health care cannot be pinpointed by science because no two human beings are exactly alike. Not only that, we as individuals are all always evolving. We are constantly moving goalposts.

This is where I believe the work becomes spiritual in nature. "Spiritual" can mean different things to different people, but to me, spiritual ultimately speaks to your relationship to yourself. Your "spirit" is the you that is having the experience. The you that is thinking the thought, the you that is moving the body, the you that is feeling the emotions. It is your inner self, your inner knowing, even your inner critic.

I believe we each find this inner connection in our own ways. It could be through creating art, music, or food. It could be through your faith, your relationship to the divine—which might register as God or the vast universe or the land itself. It could be through acts and moments of love, of awe, even of grief and of heartbreak.

How could there possibly be one reigning prescription to heal us when we feel disconnected from our very selves? It's impossible. And I think this is why there can be no "cure" for mental illness. I think this is why even when you might have a medication that works for you during one season of your life, at a certain point the remedy needs to evolve. Because you have evolved.

Being in therapy was a life raft when I felt like I was drowning. It provided me a space and taught me the language to look within, to find myself, my repressed trauma, and my uninvestigated pain. I didn't understand what I had been holding onto for my entire life, which I had instinctively done out of survival. Repression is a reflex, after all, not a conscious choice. Especially as a child, I never consciously chose to tuck away the weight of fear, anxiety, and panic so that I would always need to carry it with me.

Therapy was the life raft that pulled me out of the choppy waters, but it was me that had to find my way to the shore, step out of the life raft, and ground into my truth.

That's the work that people talk about when they say you need to "do the work." It's not just going to the therapy sessions or the healing sessions or the acupuncture, cold plunge, hot yoga, meditation, or retreat in Bali. The work is the in between. The work is when you're just with you. It's the listening, feeling, grieving, raging. It's the application of consciousness to that which you have not accepted or even been aware of. It's the steps you take from this newly exposed place.

And it is precisely because there is no separation between the mind and the body that what I was psychologically holding onto manifested into explosions of physical symptoms, when my physical self changed so dramatically. From the visible physical changes of pregnancy and postpartum, for me punctuated by surgery—a literal slicing of my very center—to the hormonal changes to the unseen but deeply felt spiritual changes . . . everything was changed. I was changed.

Whether it's baby blues or a full-blown postpartum crisis, a mother's mental health needs to be addressed and followed up on in the same way that her vaginal tears or cesarian scar are checked. We are not meant to be able to do everything and know everything and there are times when we need more help. Becoming a mother is most certainly one of those times.

If such care were normalized and encouraged, how much more well would mothers feel? How much more joy could they experience with their babies and partners? And how much more ease, love, strength, and acceptance would be created for everyone in her life?

*   *   *

For people of the global majority, there needs to also be a wider lens on the construct of Western therapy and who, and what, this model best serves. I believe that part of why families such as mine rarely discuss mental health is because there is a disconnect in language and cultural understanding. So much is lost in the diaspora.

There must have been a different way that our ancestors cared for mental health. I don't believe that our people never talked about feelings. I think their mental hygiene just looked different.

As well, those of us displaced in Western cultures have added layers of systemic trauma that we have never not been navigating, living as outsiders in systems of whiteness. If the majority of therapists are white, how comfortable and how honest could we possibly be in "unpacking" all of this invisible but ever-present oppression?

*   *   *

One of my diagnoses is PTSD—post-traumatic stress disorder. The "post" suggests that it is in the past; it's over and done with. Years after my initial diagnosis, I came across the concept of CPTSD—complex PTSD. The difference between the two is that PTSD results from a single event whereas CPTSD results from prolonged trauma. I asked my therapist if that might be what I had, as my trauma pertained to my entire childhood and relationship with my mother, not a one-off event. My therapist rejected it, as CPTSD is not officially recognized in the DSM-5, *The Diagnostic and Statistical Manual of Mental Disorders, Fifth Edition,* which is considered the main reference for mental disorders. I can't help but wonder about the impact of persistent traumatic circumstances and the need to apply a different term to describe what happens as a result.

This idea of trauma as an ongoing stress disorder has been talked about recently in the context of the genocide in Gaza. Yara M. Asi wrote in the *New York Times*: "To call what is experienced by people in Gaza today PTSD misses that these are not people in a post-trauma situation. Treatment may help a Vietnam veteran recognize that a loud sound is not always a threat. Treatment cannot help convince children in Gaza that the bombs they hear will not kill them, because the bombs might. It cannot offer comfort to a woman worried her children may starve, because they could. Rather than use the term "post-traumatic stress disorder," many have called to reframe the view of such suffering. Some have called it chronic traumatic stress disorder, and others, including Palestinian scholars, have referred to it as feeling broken or destroyed. This is not just a matter of semantics. These alternatives show that it is not enough to offer therapeutic options that place the abnormality within individuals and not within the circumstances they are experiencing. Is it not actually quite normal and understandable to feel broken or destroyed when everything you have ever known is reduced to rubble?"[17]

Asi is challenging what we understand to be disorders and whether psychological conditions are due to the person having a problem processing something or due to understandably challenging circumstances. When circumstances are dangerous and frightening, even life-threatening, isn't it a perfectly healthy response to feel traumatized?

The word trauma perhaps has become overused in popular lexicon, with the distinction often being made between little-t trauma and big-T Trauma. The thing is, just like I don't think it's an exaggeration to say that becoming a mother is traumatic, I think the experience of being human generally in and of itself is a traumatic one. Especially for those of us caught in oppressive systems of capitalism, colonialism, and racism.

I interviewed Candice Rose Valenzuela, a Black, Indigenous, Queer, and poor people allied trauma expert and mother. With an MA in both East-West Psychology and Counseling Psychology, Valenzuela lives and works at the crossroads of education, justice, and community healing. Her trauma informed analysis on Western psychology is so crucial for all of us—whether we feel we have marginalized identities or not—as we create and do the work of our healing journeys.

Valenzuela says, "I don't actually believe that any trauma is past for anyone. And I think that because of individualism in the West, we hyper focus on specific traumatic events that happened in an individual lifespan. But we disconnect those from how those events are directly related to the material conditions that we're living in right now. And I'm not just talking about poverty, I'm talking about severance from the land. I'm talking about living in a state of complete alienation from nature. Absolutely nothing is natural about how we live, whether you live in high amounts of comfort or high amounts of destitution, that spectrum is completely reliant on every part of the structure. It's not, 'oh, you're poor, your trauma never ends but I'm cool because I live in this high rise.' *Nobody's cool.* It's just, what's your access to comfort in the bullshit?

"What I've come to understand from years of study of indigenous teachings and learning from people who are much wiser than me and just my own lived experience is that the first and primary and essential traumatic event that we are all trapped in is the inception of colonialism. That's the first climate event, the first trauma event. And obviously that was a historical series of processes. But it also needs to be understood as an ongoing event that hasn't ended.

"Western psychology teaches you that your primary attachment is to your parents. I disagree. Your primary attachment is not to your parents. And so if their premise is wrong from the beginning, the healing is going to be limited because they're invested in a different perspective. Why the hell would they teach us that we actually need to heal the land if they were just going to overthrow everything? The goal of Western therapy is not for us to deeply and truly heal. It's to allow us to manage and cope our symptoms long enough to continue producing labor of whatever kind within the infrastructure and / or reducing the amount that we're able to disrupt.

"I believe our primary attachment is actually to the earth and to community. That's the home."

This collective perspective is what had been missing from my eight years of one-on-one therapy. If we are social beings, always in relationship with each other and always sharing in each others' energetic fields, then it is impossible for healing to happen in a vacuum. It also makes no sense that mental well-being would only be reserved for those who have the means to find, pay for, and have time to see a therapist.

Instead, Valenzuela asks us to consider the original severing that we all have experienced simply by virtue of living in this modern world. Our severing from the land and from each other. This is a collective trauma for us all, irrespective of our particular identities.

Valenzuela echoes what we established in the last chapter about the village: "It was never supposed to be a nuclear family. Historically, people have always existed within extended family groups. Even what we call a family is a stripped down, skeletal version that makes all the relationships so pressurized . . . how is anybody going to get that right?

Everything is dependent on you. That framing is wrong in the first place. I think that actually our parents and our social family groups are like evolutionary mechanisms to bridge or nurture the connection ultimately to the land and to one another as a collective. And because that has been ruptured, that's why you see everything you see today. And so the hyper focus on this one attachment relationship, be it your father, your mother or your significant other, I think is a way to displace those feelings and a way to keep people healing *enough*, but not actually enough to fundamentally change things."

This perspective completely challenges one of the original titles I had suggested for the book which was *Mommy Issues*. In one of my earliest therapy sessions, after my therapist had helped me see that the roots of my postpartum symptoms went much further back than the traumatic birth of my first child, I remember saying in disbelief, "I'm here because of my childhood? Because of mommy issues? Could I be more cliché?!"

And while there was and continues to be legitimate childhood trauma, *only* working within that framework limited my ability to heal. It also kept me stuck in a self-centering loop. How had *I* been wronged? How had *I* suffered? How had *I* been traumatized?

When I started to de-center my mother as the villain in my story of suffering, alongside the knowledge that recognizing my suffering was necessary and valid, it freed me to forgive. If I had inherited the blueprint of mental illness, rage, and trauma from her, she, then, must have inherited the same from her parents, all the way up through our ancestral lineage.

Incorporating Valenzuela's analysis on the loss of connection that each and every one of us feels from the land and from the collective invites us deeper into the interrogation of why we end up feeling the way we feel. This loss, this wounding, this trauma—it's spiritual. It's collective. It's not dependent on one person. As Valenzuela said—

how could anyone meet that amount of responsibility? We are all imperfect, fallible humans.

The most beautiful and alchemizing note that Valenzuela emphasizes, which brings me to tears every time I hold the truth of it, is that it's not that hurt people hurt people. No, hurt people *heal* people.

"Where would we be if hurt people weren't healing people? Everything good in this world is from hurt people that chose to heal. Western therapy is not trying to heal the suffering at all, and it's actually perpetuating it by giving you this idea that you're supposed to get rid of your trauma. You're supposed to get rid of this thing keeping you alive? Get out of here. It has anchored you in your humanity. Why would we ever want to get rid of that?"

This is exactly what I have come to realize in unpacking and processing all of the abuse, suffering, and trauma I've survived. I mean it when I say that it was all a gift. I wouldn't be me without it all.

It does require doing the work, though. It requires sitting in the muck. It requires feeling the rage and the grief. And you're not going to get it right all of the time, maybe not even most of the time. It also doesn't mean that you're going to be happy all of the time. As Valenzuela says, "We need to break the binary, colonial assumption that healing equals happy. Or that feeling distressed means I'm not healed."

So what does it mean, then, to be healed?

To me, healing is an ongoing state of being, not an end point. The goal post will always keep moving because we are always evolving. I think what matters is feeling connected to truth, your truth. You'll feel a steady resonance in that, an inner ease despite the inevitable challenges of life.

And I think it matters what we do with our hurt. May we all endeavor to be hurt people that heal people.

8

Contort

I practiced and taught yoga throughout the entirety of my first pregnancy. I thought I would be back on my mat in no time. I told my students that I expected to only be gone for about a month.

Six weeks after delivering my son via emergency cesarean, I unrolled my mat for the first time. I did not recognize the body I found myself trying to contort. Pain seared through my legs in downward dog and around my cesarean scar anytime I lengthened my belly. I could not find even a second of balance in tree pose and the simplest spinal twist felt like trying to turn a metal rod in the center of my body.

Terrified and heartbroken, I was a failure—and I was isolated from my teachers and close friends while living abroad. What's more: I was Nike's global yoga ambassador. I was supposed to have all the answers. I was supposed to bounce back. I was supposed to be recording videos of myself gliding through postnatal yoga sequences, not weeping in a fetal position.

Depression is not so neat and tidy as to have a clear starting point, but this moment when I returned to my mat for the first time postpartum was the first undone thread of my unraveling. Who was I if I didn't have my yoga practice?

*   *   *

"I have to work out every single day," my friend, a fellow mother, said, lamenting her day away from her bootcamp class. She'd spent the morning telling me about her intermittent fasting regimen and the extra weight she feared on her size-zero body. "I absolutely cannot function without exercise."

It was New Year's Day, and I instantly felt guilty about the bowl of chips I had been hovering around and hoovering up. I had been intentionally focusing on letting myself enjoy the holidays without restrictions, but I was already uncomfortable living outside of the boundaries I'd imposed on myself for most of my life. I tried not to internalize my friend's comments, as familiar as they were.

I had asked for a treadmill for Christmas when I was twelve years old. I didn't know anyone else my age who had exercise equipment on their wish list. They asked for a Caboodle or the latest Nintendo game, not for a machine that promised to fix their body.

While other teenagers joined the cheerleading team or starred in the school play, I bypassed those childish activities to work out at our local YMCA. I felt so grown-up at the time, focusing on getting as skinny as possible in order to be happy, successful, and accepted—just like the magazines told me grown women should. At five feet tall, I couldn't even properly reach the handlebars of the elliptical machines.

For decades, I was certain I could control how I felt by controlling my body. I didn't yet understand that exercise was a way to distract myself from the scary reality of my life.

*   *   *

I first found yoga through a VHS tape in the 1990s—it was an introduction to the practice led by Rodney Yee. Compared to my mother's other workout tapes featuring supermodels like Cindy

Crawford, seeing Yee—a fellow Asian person—was deeply inviting. Because Yee is a man, I watched the tape and followed along without constantly comparing my body to his. My critical mind quieted, I felt freer to focus on the movements, and I started viscerally experiencing the connection between mind and body. I always needed to be the person who knew more about exercise than anyone else. I never played any school sports but I could feel accomplished and adult by partaking in the latest fitness trends. Yoga had just started seeping into the mainstream, and I wanted to add it to my list of workouts.

I couldn't touch my toes or figure out how to avoid hyperextending my elbows. I fell out of balance poses constantly. But I was instantly hooked on the deep sense of peace and sweet fatigue that always followed Savasana—corpse pose—the final pose of any yoga practice.

I immediately started taking class every day with a teacher named Ally, who was charming, magnetic, funny, and wise without arrogance. I wanted to be more like her. It seemed obvious to me that that's what anyone who was serious about getting *good* at yoga would do. I sometimes took two classes a day. Classes were ninety minutes long and the eighty to hundred bodies in one space made the studio feel like a sauna. I walked out drenched in sweat, and I told myself I was relaxed, accomplished, enlightened, and happy.

I became more patient and less uptight. My best friend from childhood still refers to Pre-Yoga Leah and Post-Yoga Leah. And my body changed: I lost weight and I found flexibility, core strength, and steel-focused balance. I was coordinated—even graceful—on the mat. People assumed I was a dancer, which I found astonishing. I had never done anything remotely athletic or physically competitive. I loved the flattery and approval. I needed to hear more.

I became a full-time yoga teacher at twenty-four years old. By then, yoga was my life. No matter where I was or who was with me, I had to practice at least six days a week. If I missed a practice, I feared I would lose the depth and control I'd previously reached in a pose. I worried that I would feel moody and out of sorts, out of balance. The me I had meticulously marionetted would become unhinged, and everything would come crashing down.

*   *   *

It's not like I was new to feeling uncomfortable or scared—but if my world became unyoked from the careful control I was creating with my body, mind, and breath, I unconsciously feared I'd sink backward into the young, scared, child I used to be.

I had endured a childhood with an abusive and mentally ill mother. I was hit for reasons like playing piano imperfectly, objecting over being sent to a high school where I knew no one, or, in most cases, no reason at all. I lacked a reserve of motherly love to draw upon to neutralize the bad moments; there were certainly no exercises of verbal repair like we parents are taught to employ these days. But the hardest part of it all was trying to understand my mother's suicide attempts. *How could she harm herself? Why would she want to die? Does she not love us at all?*

In order to survive, I unconsciously relied on my coping mechanisms that I developed in my earliest years. I adopted an excessively extroverted personality, to the point of being voted Most Talkative in school. I was always *on*—if I could fill spaces with unsolicited stories and thoughts, there wouldn't be room for a frightening reality. *Maybe if I just acted happy all the time, that would be what was real.*

By young adulthood, I was perfectly primed for westernized yoga and its attendant new-age spiritual teachings, a prepackaged prescription promising enlightenment by way of instant gratification.

I quickly latched onto it all: *Thoughts create things. Being grateful brings you more things to feel grateful about. You'll always find peace when you center yourself on the present moment.* This was the yoga industry's rallying cry, repeated by teachers in every yoga class, among fellow yoga practitioners as we gushed about how much we loved yoga, and in books by gurus who would eventually be outed for being criminals and cult leaders.

What a relief to learn that everything was ultimately in my control. I could just think and move my way to feeling good.

If I was feeling low, I could just practice a gratitude meditation. I could sit in the stillness of being, breathing in *I am grateful for*, breathing out lists of all my blessings—names of loved ones, having food and shelter. If I wanted to manifest something, I could just visualize it, create a mood board, and say to the Universe, *Thank you in advance for bringing this to me!*

For a long while, all of this worked. I was physically and mentally well. I had the best job. I even fell in love at first sight and married my husband a few months after we met. I'd had a traumatic childhood, but I'd survived, and I was in control of my present and my future.

*   *   *

The term "spiritual bypassing" was coined in 1984 by John Welwood, a psychologist who integrated Western psychology and Buddhist spirituality. In an interview with Tricycle: *The Buddhist Review*, Welwood said, "I noticed a widespread tendency to use spiritual ideas and practices to sidestep or avoid facing unresolved emotional issues, psychological wounds, and unfinished developmental tasks. When we are spiritually bypassing, we often use the goal of awakening or liberation to try to rise above the raw and messy side of our humanness before we have fully faced and made peace with it. We may also use our notion of absolute truth to disparage or dismiss relative human needs, feelings, psychological problems, relational difficulties, and developmental deficits."[1]

As Gabriela Picciotto, PhD, explained in the *Journal of Spirituality on Mental Health*, spiritual bypassing can cause the following negative consequences: "anxiety, blind allegiance to leaders, codependency, control problems, disregard for personal responsibility, emotional confusion, excessive tolerance of unacceptable or inappropriate behavior, feelings of shame, and spiritual narcissism."[2]

While I thought I was connecting more deeply with who I was, I was actually forcing a template of truth by way of Patanjali and pranayama, further burying a past that would eventually insist on its reckoning.

* * *

My mother had her own spirituality through which she attempted to bypass her mental illness: devout Catholicism. She went to church daily, did charitable work, made donations, and prayed constantly. God would make everything better. God would reward her devotion and heal her from all her symptoms that worried and scared us all.

She continued to be unwell. No wonder she felt driven to suicide, being stuck in the false cycle of thinking that she could control her mental illness by being a good Catholic. She did what she was supposed to, and God didn't save her.

In my twenties, I sat at dinner with my family, and my mother, who was going through a particularly dark period, sat across from me. Her eyes were empty, her mood heavy. She had no appetite.

When the food arrived, I tried to encourage her to eat a little. I took bites and told her how delicious it was. I reasoned that she would feel better if she ate. She just sat there, lifeless.

"Come on, Mom, we're so lucky to be able to come to a restaurant and have good food. You have so much to be grateful for. You can't waste all this food. There are children starving in Africa!" I said.

I'll never forget the way my mom's eyes shifted from their vapid vacancy to focus squarely on mine, morphing into an icy stare.

"You just don't understand."

*   *   *

The panic attacks began shortly after we moved to New York City, when my son was one and a half years old. They always hit me when I least expected: walking in the powder of our first snowfall, getting a completely painless and routine dental cleaning, closing my eyes to go to sleep at night.

I would suddenly notice that I felt *off*. I would check in—what was wrong? Was I in pain? Was I sensing a threat I couldn't see? Was I in actual danger?

When I couldn't find any logical explanation, and especially if I tried to deny what I was feeling, my internal alarm became more insistent. My heart rate quickened, my breath caught, my stomach started to churn. I felt the uncontrollable need to run.

My panic attacks left me permanently ill-at-ease and always wondering when the next one was coming. And when the next one did come, it would compound my existing state of dread until I could no longer remember how I had moved through the world before. It was like being in a constant brace position, just waiting for inevitable impact.

I told myself I wasn't getting enough exercise. I needed to get back to practicing yoga all the time. My energy felt stagnant, I was out of sorts, I was unhappy with my body, I needed to work harder. I just needed to release more endorphins.

So I did what I had always done: more, more, more. I manically went to harder and hotter yoga classes, bootcamp classes, supercharged Pilates classes, and even trampoline classes. It was as if I thought I could beat myself into feeling okay.

What I understand in hindsight is that my lifelong coping mechanisms were no match for the literal, physical, and hormonal changes I was experiencing postpartum. Psychiatrist Pyravin Abbasova explained, "Childbirth is very different from anything else so when we cope with difficult situations in life such as emotional and psychological situations, there are coping mechanisms that help us go through, it even childhood trauma. These are events that have already happened versus when you give birth, you are still in the hormonal and physiological shift. Your body is just wrecked. No amount of coping can help you if you are not given the proper opportunity to heal your physical body which in western culture we're not. It's not even acknowledged that we need time to heal. We don't have support for at least the first forty days, someone really helping us with the baby so we just can rest, we can heal, and we can just put our bodies back together. This is where therapy really fails women because women get postpartum depression and the therapist is trying to figure out their emotions, when what we need to also understand is that the physical body is just a mess. You can say anything you want to yourself in your mind, but you also have got to put your body back together."

The answer continues to be in mothers resting and receiving better care, the opposite of what many of us insist on doing, which is too much, too soon, and on our own. We jump into the race of how quickly can I erase what I've been through, like the mother three days postpartum rushing down the street to preschool. Like me, on my mat less than two months postpartum, not recognizing my body—what if I had had the wisdom to know that of course I wouldn't recognize my body, that this was completely normal. What would my mental state have been had I sat with the miracle of what my body—what I—had accomplished, and met the changes with curiosity and reverence, rather than rejection?

One solution that Dr. Abbasova prescribes is quite simply, togetherness: "I think the indigenous cultures had it the best. I think there are different ways that different cultures did it, but I think all of them work. And with most of them, the emphasis was that there were other women. A lot of times they were older women who are more experienced who were helping you and teaching you how to take care of the baby. I think that's a huge thing for the nervous system. Just to be able to relax, knowing you're protected and taken care of versus when you're by yourself and your nervous system being constantly on edge."

The impact of hormonal changes is very real and all postpartum mothers experience it. It's part and parcel of birth. Physical therapist Amber Bloom, PT, MSPT had a particularly complex situation that her doctors did not catch right away: "I've always been on thyroid medication because of my hypothyroidism. My thyroid levels were monitored when I was pregnant but no one monitored them afterwards. I lost all the pregnancy weight in four weeks and I had so much anxiety, but nobody made the connection. I didn't even make the connection and I feel I should have known. It was only months later that doctors realized I had too much thyroid medication."

The disconnect within the health care system when it comes to understanding a postpartum woman's mental health can lead to suffering that can be avoided. In Bloom's case, she feels it was just an accident that her thyroid levels were not checked, but why wouldn't the effects of a prescribed medication be closely monitored? How many other postpartum women are experiencing this or similar cracks in care? At a time when new mothers are trying to find their footing in the most life-altering role, we all deserve and need better. The cost is simply too high.

*   *   *

It was during a visit to LA about a year into motherhood that I experienced my first panic attack on the mat. I was back at my home studio in Santa Monica, taking a class from one of my longtime favorite teachers when it happened. The panic expanded in my body like the water from a spilled glass spreading across a surface. I jumped up from my mat, unable to force myself to stay in place. I felt the need to run—from my mat, the studio, my very self. I was embarrassed, but the feeling of panic was stronger than my humiliation. I can't remember what I later told my teacher—maybe that I felt ill? Had an emergency with my child? Got my period?

I thought up a lot of these kinds of excuses as the panic attacks became more frequent. Putting my head down in child's pose? It would hit. Winding my arms into eagle pose? Like a slap in the face. Closing my eyes to quiet my mind? My breath froze in my throat. Sitting still to meditate? I was suffocating, the walls were closing in, the floor would collapse beneath me.

I bought a book called *Yoga for Anxiety*, thinking maybe I wasn't doing the right kind of yoga. I sought advice from friends and fellow moms at my son's school, most of whom seemed flummoxed that exercise and meditation weren't working for me like it did for them.

"What do you have to feel anxious about?" they asked. "You have everything you could ever need. Are you practicing enough self-care? Why are you dwelling on your son's birth?"

Maybe I was drinking too much coffee and not eating enough greens.

Maybe I just needed to be more grateful.

Maybe I needed to become a different person.

*   *   *

It's not lost on me that the Asian practice I initially experienced through an Asian teacher would ultimately be watered down and resold to me through the filter of whiteness. During my entire career as a yoga teacher, I did not have the racial literacy or confidence to even admit to myself that I was a token in yet another whitewashed industry, that my presence perhaps helped to legitimize a stolen spiritual practice if only by softening an otherwise pervasive whiteness. I wasn't South Asian, of course, but I ticked a diversity box.

Most famous yoga teachers and yoga influencers are white, even if they're hidden by bindi stickers, mala beads, and self-appointed Sanskrit names. When you search "yogagirl" on Instagram, the result is a blonde woman with nearly two million followers. How many Indian cover models has *Yoga Journal* had?

Yoga Alliance, the largest nonprofit association representing the international yoga community, conducted a "first of its kind global survey researching the practice and profession of yoga" and announced in November 2023 that "stress management and mental health are driving growing interest and participation, yet many underserved communities are largely left out."[3] The survey found that a significant number of people—49 percent who are existing yoga practitioners and 37 percent of the general public—were advised by a medical professional to try yoga to benefit their health.

Shannon Roche, president and CEO of Yoga Alliance, explained in the press release announcing the survey. "Scientific research has demonstrated that yoga is highly effective in helping individuals manage stress and cope with mental health conditions. As concerns about mental health and loneliness increase around the globe, the perception of yoga must shift from solely a fitness modality or hobby to a vital, low-cost, high-value self directed health intervention that can, and should, be accessible to everyone."[4]

If yoga has the potential to positively impact mental health, it is something that must be accessible to everyone. According to the survey, in 2016, 36.7 million Americans practiced yoga and in 2022, that number rose to 38.4 million Americans, spending $21 billion on the practice.[5] However, of these millions of Americans practicing yoga, there was found to be "distinct demographic inequities"[6] which cause yoga spaces to feel like white spaces rather than universal ones.

Indeed, the survey found that as of 2022, 71 percent of people practicing yoga are white, 88 percent of people teaching yoga are white, and 85 percent of yoga studio owners are white. There is also a clear socioeconomic disparity: those who practice or work in the yoga industry are more likely to have a college degree and own their home than the general public.

Roche continued, "Amid the economic contraction we see that individuals were finding the practicality and value in yoga as a way to alleviate the numerous challenges brought on by the COVID-19 pandemic. While economic growth, spending, and participation in yoga is encouraging, the research also showed that Asian, Black, and Hispanic communities in the United States are underrepresented as yoga practitioners, teachers, and studio owners. Studies have shown that these communities are less likely to have access to mental health resources, yoga studios, or similar wellness resources which make treatment more difficult. Taken together, this information offers yet another example of the systemic underinvestment in proven holistic wellness practices, like yoga, in historically marginalized communities, when these practices can often trace their roots back to these very same communities."[7]

In addition to accessibility, yoga does not always feel inviting for people of the global majority. The survey found that Asian, Black, and Hispanic people did not find the culture and lifestyle around yoga appealing and "referenced a stereotype of the average yoga practitioner being a 'fit, white woman.'"[8]

Roche concluded, "Yoga has the potential to benefit anyone who practices, but the way it is shared and/or portrayed can impede or enhance its widespread acceptance. As a yoga community, we need to be intentional in our efforts to publicly communicate and normalize the diversity of students, teachers, and practitioners that actually exist, and how yoga can aid people from all communities, regardless of race, ethnicity, income level, age, body type, ability, or gender."[9]

This study lays bare the inherent problem with the yoga and wellness world in centering a particular identity—the "fit, white woman"—to whom the practice of yoga does not belong in the first place. I think of all the women, the mothers, who are left out of this space known for its potential to support and heal. The messaging is that only a certain type of mother is worthy.

Whiteness, fueled by capitalism, has appropriated, bastardized, and commodified this ancient, sacred practice from the East. What I understand now is that my deepest sense of self was finally rejecting and revolting against continuing to buy into a world that was not made for me and therefore was not a safe space for me. No matter how many classes I took, no matter how consistently I meditated, no matter how much I contorted myself—I would always be outside of whiteness.

The thing is, whiteness harms us all, irrespective of our racial identity. It robs all of us of our true uniqueness, our ability to connect to our inner wisdom, and ultimately our humanity. The more we understand that it is the ideology of white supremacy—of any hierarchal system that categorizes people based on any particular parameters—that is the enemy and not one another, the less defensive we will be and the more connected we can become to ourselves as well as to one another.

I interviewed Lindsey Guttilla, the founder of Hudson Mind Body Spirit, a spiritual center offering classes, community, and mentorship. Guttilla is an intuitive healer, end-of-life doula, yoga and meditation teacher, mother—and she is white.

"The reason I started the center was because I felt like I had been so harmed by the spiritual world. I was misled and harmed by teachers and cult-like practices. I realized there's so much bullshit in the spiritual world that is perpetuating white supremacy and the colonization of these practices. And I thought about other people taking classes who hadn't realized the truth of this spiritual world— the spiritual industrial complex. I want to be a part of this world and be of service without harming people in the process.

"I've had direct experiences with different power dynamics including sexual abuse and harm with my own teachers, both female and male. I felt very much like something was missing. Especially in America, I believe what's missing is community. We are sort of this cultureless society and there's just no community dynamic. I recognize that even as we were trying in the spirituality and yoga space to emulate structures of community, care, service, and growth, there's no actual support of any type of community structure. That's why, for example, the whole guru thing doesn't work in Western society.

"For me, the work is teaching people how to spot spiritual bypassing, how to spot these systems of harm, and then also how to cultivate this connection outside of any other practice that they've been taught or sold. It is my purpose and my mission to expose that side of the world and then to help people understand what it actually means to do the inner work. How to make your own authentic practice that is aligned with you and your soul. That is your own unique thing. It has to be real. It can't be performative. It has to be something that you actually turn to in times of chaos, in times of need, in times of joy. It has to be an embodied connection.

"This is what I try to teach people. I hope to teach discernment and a sense of agency which means it's your responsibility to question everything. To not hold anyone on a pedestal, to use their own inner guidance system, to not dismiss that quiet voice within, those little inner nudges. And how do we do that? Through meditation, through prayer. Prayer is what I would call the language of the soul. And that is a very subjective experience for each person. But that is the way to know what is right. Because everyone is intuitive. Everyone that has a soul and a body can really tune in and know what is right for them."

Guttilla experienced harm in the wellness world, even as a white woman. She recognized that the lack of community, discernment, and connection to the real work paved the way for spiritual bypassing, which leaves all of us vulnerable. What Guttilla offers through her work is a way back to ourselves. The answer is always within, which can feel both liberating and overwhelming, but any spiritual work is made much worse by self-proclaimed teachers, healers, and leaders who themselves are not doing the inner work and instead playing into systems of capitalism and white supremacy.

Yoga, meditation, and other holistic practices are naturally where many mothers turn for their mental health. We have been sold the idea that these practices will help us feel more grounded, more centered, and more balanced. And many of us do learn useful techniques rooted in deep breathing, presence, and mindfulness—all of which help soothe the nervous system. But there is an inherent shallowness because the yoga industry here in the west is severed from its roots in the east. It's been captured by those who espouse and best represent Western and therefore white supremacist ideals, from the clothes that are worn, the size of our bodies, the color of our skin, and how much money is in our bank account. We have gotten to a point where the lines of spirituality and ego have become blurred and tangled together.

So when a mother finds herself truly struggling—isolated, desperate, and afraid, how could such a vapid and vain space provide her the community and healing she is looking for?

*　　*　　*

For decades, I tried to contort myself into something I was not: white, unaffected, controlled, free. Of course, I was never in control. Things happen that are random, unfair, and senseless—and it's not because I didn't try hard enough, think positively enough, or drink enough cold-pressed juice. It certainly wasn't because I had bad karma. But I kept trying to manifest, meditate, and force my way out of it all; I kept trying to control my symptoms of depression, anxiety, and panic with self-flagellation. And I did my best to contort myself into a world that wasn't based in reality: No matter how deeply I breathed, I could not breathe out my trauma, my childhood, my pain, my desires.

Yoga and meditation had worked for me for a long time, but when it was time for my demons to truly be unearthed and contended with, trying to do it all by myself with my practice was not enough. I could not will my way out of suffering.

The answer was not to do more, to beat myself into submission, to force myself into manufactured wellness spaces, manicured mom groups, or clothing that no longer fit. The answer was to slow down and to face myself and to do the work—to see myself for who I really was, perhaps for the first time ever—and to fully accept myself.

I heard once that if you're having a lucid nightmare, particularly a recurring one in which you're being chased, instead of running away, you should stop and face that which you are running from. Assume there is a message your subconscious has for you. Ask what it is you are meant to learn. Listen.

I started sitting with my feelings and my fear in this way. I started listening to my body when it communicated to me: When I felt panic rise while taking a yoga class, I gave myself permission to step off the mat, even if I felt embarrassed. When I felt the weight of anxiety at bedtime, I allowed myself to watch a comedy, in the same way that I might distract my child from his fear of the flu shot by making him laugh.

I learned that I needed to practice more gentleness and ease with myself. I was running on empty, running away from myself, running myself down. Once I stopped trying to bypass my pain, I could hear what needed to be expressed, processed, and healed. Only then could I start to ask for help to move forward with steadiness toward freedom.

I still deeply value my yoga practice, which I have finally parsed free from the yoga industry, from the spiritual industrial complex. I still believe there is something magical about the union of intention, body, and breath. But my panic attacks were nudges from my body's inherent wisdom—just as much as the Savasana highs were. I understand now that my path to wellness and joy are not through self-punishment or devotion to an industry that largely does not welcome my whole self. Then—as now—my body knows that there is so much more to understand about what I have held onto—my unexamined pain from childhood and more—so that I can work to release it.

9

Mixed

"Hey, come here, I have to tell you something," I say to my husband, motioning for him to lean in. He lowers his head toward me. Laughing, I whisper into his ear, "I'm the only *yellow* person here!"

We are having a big family dinner at his parents' home in England. My husband's mother is English and his father is Irish. He has two siblings who have married fellow British people. His brother's wife is part English and part Pakistani and I have always felt an innate camaraderie in her presence, but, I am the only non-white person in the family. Even my kids, of course, are part white.

My husband looks back at me uncomfortably, unsure of how to respond. *Was I joking? Should he joke back? Was I upset? Was there anything he could do to fix the situation?* He later tells me that nobody else was thinking about me being the only Asian person at the table, let alone thinking of me as "yellow."

*　*　*

I moved from Hong Kong to London about a month after my husband and I met on a Nike set in Santa Monica. We hardly knew each other but neither of us wanted to attempt to do long distance. We'd both had long-term relationships that had fallen apart and we'd both been through health scares in the year or so before we had met. We were in our thirties and we were honest and vulnerable with each other about where we wanted to go in life: a partner, kids, a beautiful home, and adventures. Our values felt aligned and we both felt an instant spark of commitment to each other.

I landed at Heathrow with all of the belongings I'd accumulated through my adult life as a yoga teacher. As my future tall, British husband walked toward me, it felt like I had stepped into that airport scene from *Love Actually*. He held my hand the whole way into the city on the Heathrow Express.

I moved into a makeshift loft/art studio that he was sharing with friends: two married couples. Coincidentally, we girls were all American and the boys were all British. Everyone, but me, was affiliated to the art world. Everyone, but me, was white. I felt like I didn't belong, but this was a feeling I was familiar with.

I grew up in California, but despite all its supposed diversity, I still grew up as a racialized minority. I still grew up as an outsider in the system of white supremacy. I didn't have the language for this at the time, but I felt it. Children feel these kinds of truths in their bones. And it's constantly confirmed by the media, by teasing and ridicule ("just" "microaggressions"), by our own parents' biased opinions, and for Asians in particular, by being made to feel invisible.

The first time it occurred to me that I was the only non-white person alongside my husband at the dinner table was on my very first night in London. Giles and my new roommates were preparing a roast dinner. I had never had a roast before! As is the case with a lot of Asian families, I didn't grow up having roast turkey on holidays. We had a precooked, store-bought Honeybaked ham and instant mashed potatoes out of a box alongside Korean dishes.

It felt wonderfully festive to see everyone take on a task for my first-ever roast. Hilary was peeling carrots, Graham was dousing chunks of potato with duck fat (which he would only reveal to me later, as he feared I, being a health-conscious yogi with a yet to be diagnosed eating disorder, wouldn't have eaten them otherwise), Val minced garlic and lamented that her fingers would now smell like garlic for days, Sam poured everyone drinks, and Giles prepared the turkey. I was quietly relieved that everyone insisted that I just sit and relax after such a long haul flight from the East because I would have had no idea how to help with such a Western feast. I felt so out of my comfort zone.

Another couple joined us for dinner. I looked around and counted seven white people and myself. The token person of color. The only yellow person at the table.

This was a scene that repeated itself countless times through my five years living in London. It's not that London is not racially diverse. According to Gov.UK, the 2021 Census data reported that London was the most ethnically diverse region in England and Wales, with 46.2 percent of Londoners identifying as Asian, Black, mixed, or "other" ethnic groups.[1] And these kinds of numbers will be cited as evidence that we are in a post-racial world. But such demographics don't take into account who continues to be in power. Who is most represented in media. Who dictates culture.

There was one occasion when we sat down to watch a movie that Giles had watched as a child: *The Pink Panther* starring Peter Sellers as Inspector Clouseau. We were all laughing at its slapstick, over-the-top humor and ridiculousness.

But the film, like much media, is rife with racism. Inspector Clouseau has an Asian sidekick/servant named Cato Fong. He is a stereotypically Asian character, that is, very good at martial arts. Inspector Clouseau repeatedly refers to him as "my little yellow friend."

I quietly flinched every time I heard that phrase uttered. I told myself: *This is from a different time, a more racially ignorant time. Nobody is calling ME their little yellow friend. This is just a silly movie with people acting ridiculous and saying ridiculous things.* I said nothing in order to avoid any awkwardness. I tried to push away the thought, "Does anyone else realize this is blatantly disparaging to Asian people?"

My guess is that most people don't notice or take seriously these harmful stereotypes. And that is precisely the problem. It has always been just normal, even if unconsciously so, to hear us being portrayed as Other, as Less Than.

The fact is, *The Pink Panther* franchise was hugely popular, which means countless people heard and probably went on to repeat the phrase, "my little yellow friend." We all grew up with media portraying Asian people—*my* people—in a dehumanizing way. One might argue that things were different back then, that we are all so much more aware and less racist now. But, are we?

And since "white" is broadly used to describe people from Europe and "Black" is used to describe people from Africa and the Caribbean, one might wonder why it's not okay to attribute "yellow" to people from Asia. "Yellow," along with "red" to refer to Indigenous peoples of America, was historically used in disparaging ways. Describing Asian people as "yellow" does not come from a place of inclusivity or equality. It comes from the pejorative terms "yellow peril" or "yellow terror" or "yellow specter," which aimed to portray people from Asia as dangerous, threatening, and alien to the Western world.

*   *   *

The reality of my racial trauma became undeniable once I became a mother. I used to think this was due to worrying how other people might view me—as the help, as a green card wife, as a foreigner—but reflecting on it now, I think it had just as much to do with my own battle of internalized self-rejection.

I still travel with my children's birth certificates and our marriage certificate, tying our Irish last name to my Korean maiden name. Despite the fact that we all have the same legal surname, there is a part of me that worries that my very identity as their mother will be questioned. Will I be believed? Am I seen as human enough?

I worry about how life will be for my children, growing up as a racialized minority. But they are neither Asian nor white—they're both.

My son is always trying to make sense of this.

"Am I . . . tan?" he asked one summer, investigating the color of his forearm.

"Well, yes, you are, but, that doesn't describe your race."

"Then what's my race?"

"You're mixed."

"But what color is that?"

It's a good question, one that I struggle to find a sensible answer to.

My four-year-old daughter is also already trying to understand her identity. I overheard her ask her dad the other night while brushing her teeth, "Am I Asian?"

"Yes, you are, you're Korean."

"But you're not Korean, right?"

"No, I'm white."

"Am I white?"

"Yes, you're Korean and you're white—you're English and you're Irish. You're mixed!"

As they themselves try to get a grasp of their mixed identities, I wonder how they will be seen by peers, teachers, and society at large. I am grateful to live in the so-called melting pot of New York City, where it is the norm to see a truly diverse mix of fellow humans.

My kids get ramen and kimchi at their school cafeteria, something unthinkable when I was of school age.

But there are still concerning situations, such as my son being the one kid consistently singled out if there is a group disturbance in a class, being the one that is made to write an apology letter to the white kid but not vice versa. Is this due to systemic racism? I can't know for sure because I'm never there in the moment—maybe my son was the one centrally at fault—but it's a valid question that plagues many of us parents of color.

Even at my daughter's Two's preschool, racism rears its ugly head.

One afternoon, she was home dancing around and she started pulling at the corners of her eyes.

"Don't I look funny? I look so funny like this!"

I was taken aback. "Why are you doing that to your eyes?"

"John told me to do it. He says I look funny with eyes like this."

John is a blond, blue-eyed boy. He would have been three years old at the time, so, was it simply a random coincidence that he was telling an Asian child to pull her eyes into a famously racist stereotype about Asian people? Again, I can't know for sure, but I know what my gut tells me.

*   *   *

My pointing out my "yellow-ness" at a table of white people was perhaps an immature way of expressing discomfort and the desire to belong; an unsophisticated attempt to reclaim a word that has historically been used to tokenize and stereotype my people. Wasn't I everyone's little yellow friend? The proof was right there on the TV screen in the form of a supposedly harmless, silly film.

It was a protective reflex: Let me offend myself before I can be offended by anyone else.

The actual hue of my skin is not really yellow at all. At the height of a New York City summer, my skin is tanned brown. In the wintertime, my skin is paler, closer to the color of my husband's and my children's, closer to white than yellow.

But nobody would ever describe or see me as white.

And everyone—*everyone*—sees color.

As parents, whatever our racial identities, it is our responsibility to raise race-conscious kids, especially those of us living in white societies. It is not good enough and in fact it is untrue and harmful to claim to simply not see skin color. Feeding a false veneer of equality actually perpetuates the power of systemic racism. We continue to see race-driven hate crimes. There is so much work to be done in seeking racial equality and equity—in seeking liberation for all identities. It needs to be understood that discriminatory treatment is not only found in the extreme actions of hate groups and that microaggressions are still just acts of racism. We need to have the uncomfortable conversations in the big and the small ways, in our families and in our communities.

Raising my biracial son and daughter in a society hostile to their very existence—just last year, Senator Mike Braun of Indiana said that the Supreme Court was wrong to repeal bans on interracial marriage[2]—presents thorny issues for me *and* my marriage. My white, British husband and I both come from insular cultures that prize purity, and in a way, it was an act of rebellion to choose each other. Our partnership is built on a deep love and a desire for our personal choices to dismantle dominant systems. But, still, we clash sometimes. Thirteen years in, he still sometimes forgets to take his shoes off in the house. We struggle to communicate the nuances of our backgrounds to each other—and even when we can get the point across, there can be friction.

It's critical to us that we honor our children's dual identities: Korean American and British. But it can create an uncomfortable distance: I'm in charge of the Korean piece, he's in charge of the British component. It leaves us focusing on separate things—things we cannot easily grasp about each other.

Conversations around identity, race, and racism continue to challenge our marriage. I can end up feeling frustrated and resentful when my husband does not immediately understand why I might be triggered by something, such as the night we happened to be watching a cooking show about a white chef who had become famous for his ramen.

"Why do we have to watch these white dudes making ramen?" I quipped.

My husband had been unwinding to the hum of the television after a particularly stressful day at work and he was caught off guard by my sudden sarcasm. He had put that show on because we both enjoy cooking shows.

"God, can't we just watch anything in peace? He's a chef who lived in Japan! Why can't he talk about ramen?"

"Don't you know food appropriation when you see it?"

"Spare me your lectures, yes, I know what food appropriation is. Not everything is appropriation. It isn't appropriation every time a white person makes ramen. You just cooked Italian pasta!"

"Me cooking at home is not the same as someone who gets to rise through the system and end up on Netflix! I'm tired of seeing white people getting all the opportunities! It's systemic racism! I want to hear about ramen from a Japanese person, who can talk about the culture, the history! I can't believe you're defending someone you don't even know!"

"You have such a chip on your shoulder! It's just a cooking show!"

"It's not *just* a cooking show! It's indicative of how white supremacist this world is! Don't you care? You have Asian children!"

It took several days before we could revisit the conversation. I was stuck on the fact that if I had made that first comment to any one of my friends who is not white, it would not have gone that way. They would have responded in kind, perhaps offered their own sarcastic appraisal, we would maybe have rolled our eyes and moved on. My husband was stuck on the fact that it was 11:00 p.m. on a work day and he was just trying to watch something relaxing, could I maybe not go into one of my righteous diatribes, just this once?

To me, it felt like he was taking my comment personally. I wasn't talking about HIM, why was he getting so mad? Why was it seeming like he was defending and upholding white supremacy?

To him, it felt like I was unaware that he was overwhelmed and tired, why couldn't I just let him have some space?

It's hard to come from such different lived realities, to be seen and treated so differently by the world. I think sometimes there can be resentment. For me, it's only over the last few years that I have really come to understand my internalized racism and have finally shed the impossible but lifelong wish to be white. There is such heartbreak and anger in realizing the time I lost to not accepting myself. These emotions can rise unexpectedly and whoever is around might get caught in the crossfire. I of course don't blame my husband for being white or for my not being white. But my anger at injustice and my worry about how our kids will be impacted by a world that will never see them as white—that's all very real and very valid.

Perhaps the messiness and miscommunication are part of the process. Coming from different cultural identities necessitates an openness to learning and an acceptance that the other person isn't always going to get it . . . and how could they? But we can keep inviting each other in. We can keep asking questions. We can keep listening.

We can—and must—keep breaking down systems of racial hierarchy, and it matters that we endeavor to do this within our own homes.

I constantly contend with all of this as a mother to our mixed kids. How do I protect them from the internalized racism I carried with me for too long? How do I teach them about the way of the world without making them angry, resentful, or fearful? How different is their concept of their identity from that of mine, considering they are neither fully Asian nor fully white?

Writer and mother Joon Ae Haworth-Kaufka relates to the feeling of growing pains when it comes to grappling with questions of identity in the context of her mixed-race family: "These kids hold so much. And whether we like it or not, they hold the tensions of our relationships with our white partners. For me, being a woman of color who is committed to liberation—in the world, in my community, and in myself, being partnered with a white cis man means to be immersed in the good struggle of constantly undoing and becoming within the context of my own relationship. When I undo, and when I become, I change my relationship to whiteness, and therefore my partnership changes. Sometimes this is wonderful and sometimes it is very difficult. People change at different paces and we can change together as well as apart. And—our kids are not separate from us."

"It can't be easy to be the partially-European mixed-kid of a fiery, politically conscious activist mother. In their bodies and souls, they have inherited the racial trauma of us and of our ancestors as well as the trauma of white colonizer violence. My kids have to listen to me constantly talking about whiteness—and my disgust for it. No matter how much I have tried to tell them that this is not about *white skin*, but about *whiteness* as a cultural construct of racial supremacy within a socially constructed hierarchy of power and privilege, I can't imagine that they wouldn't *not* internalize that they are a part of and are privileged by a system of violence.

"On the other hand, mixed kids still experience racism—and the extent is how white passing they are. And if we're raising them with a critical eye, they see whiteness in their white parent, too. They develop the ability to have a sharp racial analysis of what is happening inside their own homes. All of this is hard!

"I always tell my white husband, I do this work because I LOVE the world! I love life! I love freedom. And so it is extremely painful to experience racism in this world that I love so, so much, and it is even more painful to come home to the place that is supposed to be my sanctuary from the world's harms and see the same things reflected in my home life, in my relationship with my life partner, one of the people I love more than anyone in the world. And then it's even more intense to have to confront this fear that I have that it is possible for my own children, people I love more than anyone ever, to internalize racism both as the receiver *and* as the perpetrator."

Admittedly, I had not yet considered what it means for my mixed kids to understand and contend with *their* whiteness. Do they feel like they belong in all spaces or in none? Are there enough mixed-race kids in their world that this will not be so much of an issue for them at least in their day to day? Am I mothering them in a way that honors all parts of their identity without emphasizing one over the other? How do I help them understand that while they are people of the global majority, they also carry the privilege of whiteness in their identity?

I love Haworth-Kaufka's advice: "I think, in part, some of the work we must do with our kids is to help facilitate spaciousness. I think this is the potential that is beautiful. These kids potentially have the capacity to hold so much, and this is a good thing. Not to ask them to bear the weight of things, but to hold space for them to have a lot of inner complexity and the potentiality for immense compassion. Just imagine how expansive their inner worlds have the potential to be."

I think this is something that my husband and I can do together for our children. We already understand the complexity of being in an interracial marriage and the challenges our differences bring to our family dynamic. If we can commit to approaching each other with curiosity, not only can we set a powerful example for our son and daughter, but I think we can find our own inner healing.

I asked therapist, mother, and transracial, transnational adoptee Alisha Bennett about her experience raising her mixed raced—Korean and Jewish—daughter. Born in Korea, Bennett was adopted by a white family in Michigan, in a predominantly white community with no one that looked like her except for other Korean adoptees, also adopted into all white families.

The issue of identity has always loomed large for Bennett although she has reclaimed her Korean identity as an adult. By the time she had her daughter, Bennett was already deeply proud of her Korean roots, a pride that her young daughter has inherited and learned: "We talk to Coco about how she does have these European roots but she's like, I'm Korean. Sometimes at the dinner table, she'll say, 'Mom, me and you are Korean, but Dad's not.' She just loves being Korean. She loves being in Korean school. She's always asking our Korean tutor to teach her words in Korean. She loves to wear her 한복—*hanbok* (traditional Korean clothes). She loves her mixed-race Korean babysitter whom she calls 언니—*unnie* (older sister). She asks, 'When are we going back to Korea?' She is fully embracing her Korean-ness.

"I was very intentional about this. I have made very conscious, intentional efforts of integrating her identity and our customs into her life. There are layers of complication for me because I've realized that there is so much that I was not taught. I didn't know Koreans celebrated lunar new year until recently. No one fucking taught me that."

I understand so deeply what Bennett means when she says that there are layers of complication, although she has even more to hold as an adoptee. The severing in her case has been quite literal. But I am so in awe of the work she has done to heal and to continue to heal. I love that she proudly says that she is in her *self-love era.* I can only imagine how liberating it must be for her daughter to have been brought into this world with a mother who is determined to be a living example of accepting and celebrating yourself.

Both of our daughters are still young, but what I have been able to observe about each of them at this stage is an exuberance in expressing themselves, an ease in their bodies, a joie de vivre. And while I am truly so happy—and relieved—that mothers like Bennett and me are able to guide our children down better paths of self-acceptance than we found ourselves on in our own childhoods, recognizing how differently I grew up is painful. I can't help but feel grief for what I did not have as I do my best to give just that to my children.

This grief, holding the hollowness of what never was, is part of the healing. It can feel scary to face; we may fear that we won't be able to handle the avalanche of emotions, tears, and aching—all of which I have experienced in writing this chapter. I think it's why this chapter has been the hardest for me to write. But I am sure that feeling the pain is part of the healing.

If we think back to generational trauma being the inheritance of both the bad as well as the good, we know that the bad *and* the good, the trauma *and* the tools to heal are necessarily interwoven. We know that when we heal ourselves, we are changing the relationships we have with others—past, present, and future.

I believe this means that we are also healing our past selves. We are healing our inner child.

I can't change history. I can't ever have had a mother who was available to mother me. Bennett cannot go back to her first three months of life before she was taken from her birth mother and from her motherland. But we can sit with those versions of ourselves. Maybe that's why genes make it so that children end up looking like their parents. So that when we look at our children, we see traces of ourselves. Maybe when we are doing our best to parent our children, we are also sending that care to our child selves.

I look at both of my kids, who both my husband and I agree look more Korean than they do mixed race, and as their mother, I of course think they are incredibly adorable, perfect even. Sometimes my son and I will be at the mirror together and he will exclaim, "I look exactly like you!" And he says it joyfully, not with any criticism or rejection, the way many people of the global majority have often looked at ourselves. Through my children I am seeing beyond my once-perceived flaws. I am stepping into my self-love era.

10

Shatter

"I'm going to punch you in the face!"

That's what I said to eight-year-old Ryker while we were picking up our rental car at LAX. I said it loudly. Several staff members heard me, a nearby father heard me, my husband heard me, and my son, of course, heard me. I had said it inches away from his face, seething with anger, fists clenched at my sides.

We had just flown over from NYC. It was only our second flight since pre-Covid and my anxiety had been working overtime as we were starting to re-enter the world outside of the protective bubble I'd insisted we all stay in for the previous two years. The process of deplaning and picking up your rental car at LAX is painfully inefficient. It's a lot of waiting, a lot of whining, a lot of wishing you had a coffee but how could you possibly hold one more thing?

Despite having pre-requested a toddler car seat for my two-year-old, we were given an infant's car seat. So, a staff member took us to a storage closet and the doors opened to stacks and stacks of plastic-wrapped car seats of varying brands and sizes, none that seemed suitable for our daughter.

Impatient and frustrated, my son stood right in front of me, tugging my arm, asking one question after another:

Why don't they have the same car seat we have?

Why can't she use this car seat?

Why do babies have to ride backwards?

What happens if a baby doesn't ride backwards?

Did I ride backwards?

Why didn't we just bring our car seat?

How much longer is this going to take?

Can we go now?

And on and on and on and on.

I promise you that until my hinges came off, I was implementing and saying what all the parenting experts and books advise:

Hey bud, grownups are talking right now, you need to wait.

I can see you're feeling frustrated right now. I am too. It would be really helpful if you could give me a second to figure this out.

I understand you have some questions. I will explain it all to you later. Right now, I need to focus on finding the right car seat for your sister.

Okay, that's enough. You need to stop.

Please, be quiet.

Go sit over there with your dad and sister.

Go, now.

I said, go! Stop talking! Stop grabbing my shirt!

I'm going to punch you in the face!

My son finally went quiet. He looked back at me in shock, in total disbelief. I could see people out of my periphery. I'm pretty sure that that other father clutched his child a little tighter, buckled him into his (appropriately sized) car seat, and sped out of my poisonous parenting radius.

I caught my husband's eye. He was shaking his head with a mixture of disappointment and disgust. I knew what he would say to me:

You're the adult.

You need to de-escalate the situation, not make it worse.

You have anger issues.

I wasn't so consumed by my emotions that I couldn't see that I had gone too far. I was immediately embarrassed, if not instantly ready to take accountability.

My son got out of my face, I found a car seat, and we were finally ready to get going.

"Ryker, I'm sorry I shouted at you. I'm sorry I said I was going to punch you in the face. I would never punch you in the face. I should not have said that."

"Okay," he quietly mumbled.

"Mommy is not a robot. I don't have endless patience. It's not okay that you were interrupting me. You made a difficult situation more difficult."

"Okay."

"Still, I should not have said that to you. I'm sorry. I am never going to say that to you again."

Later, my husband and I would have an argument about what happened. I kept defending myself, saying, "But I didn't actually punch him in the face!"

*   *   *

You have anger issues. You have such a short fuse. You have the Korean temper. You are so fiery.

I have heard these things on and off throughout my life. My boyfriend in college practically shed a tear at a New Year's Eve dinner with friends one year when I shared that my resolution was to be more patient . . . God, was I *that* bad?

I didn't *feel* like an angry, fiery person. Sure, I would get irritated or frustrated from time to time, but who didn't? And it always seemed to be in response to something that wasn't fair or right: a rude salesperson, a classmate spreading a rumor, things not going perfectly to plan. Surely it was normal to feel angry in these moments?

Looking back, I wonder how much of the criticism around my anger was actually about me and how much of it was buying into and perpetuating the societal expectation that women—particularly Asian women—should not be expressing anger? The stereotype of the meek and subservient Asian woman is well-known, juxtaposed with the character of the dragon lady—strong and powerful but in a deceitful way. Neither are meant to be flattering and both stereotypes assume a hypersexualization of Asian women.

But the people in my life were indeed accurately observing the quickness and intensity with which I would become consumed with anger—literally enraged. I had never been taught that anger was a valid human emotion and I had certainly never been taught how to appropriately understand and process anger. As a child, I had been on the receiving end of my mother's chaotic, undeserved anger and I had in turn suppressed my own anger at how I was treated, a necessary coping mechanism to preserve whatever safety I did have. The thing with coping mechanisms is that they become absorbed into our personality, and we automatically defer to them as habitual responses long after the threat that created them has passed. So, in any anger-inciting situation, it was as if my brain and body were back in my childhood. I did not know how to safely respond, I was too afraid to be confrontational, so my anger would compound. I would find myself fuming, unable to move on from the moment. Frequently, my anger would be more noticeable in my body and in silent facial expressions than in anything I was able to verbalize. In that way, perhaps it felt that much more uncontrolled, unhinged, even childish.

*   *   *

Shortly after we returned from LA, my childhood best friend was in town with her husband. We all went out for brunch together. As expected, my daughter was her sweet and amenable self, happy to eat and be entertained by grownups while my son was endlessly unrelaxing to have around. He kept making smart aleck remarks and jokes that were more mean than funny.

My friend just chuckled and said, "Ryker, there's nothing you could say that would surprise me. You're just like your mommy! She was just as fiery as you are!"

I wasn't surprised to hear my friend say this as I'd heard it many times before, but something hit me differently this time. I heard a small voice within me say, "Well, imagine if you had had the childhood I had, you'd be fiery too."

I could suddenly see the connection between my short fuse and what I had endured as a child. It had been terrifying to grow up in my home—a mother with bipolar/manic depression who would morph from being catatonically unavailable to physically and emotionally abusive, shrieking STA-CCA-TO from the kitchen, and when I did not hit the piano keys with the appropriate pressure and tempo, come storming through the house to hit me repeatedly in the head. If she happened to be holding a utensil, she would also hit my hands as my fingers desperately tried to strike the right keys, in the right way, not daring to stop playing even as I started bleeding, willing my tears to fall silently and stealthily. Hearing me cry would only make her more violent.

* * *

Summer ended, and the school year started for my children. I continued to be triggered by my son's behavior. He would not listen. He would goad me. He would emphatically do the opposite of what I asked. Every morning became a recurring battle. Where was the ONE

T-shirt that he absolutely had to wear on THIS day? Why hadn't I gotten the EXACT cereal he just HAD to have? Why did he even have to go to school?

Morning after morning, I would end up roaring at him. I mean, actually roaring. I wouldn't hit him, but I felt the rage inside. Rage that could easily propel regrettable actions. My daughter would stand by shell-shocked, my dog would bark maniacally, sometimes nipping at me, overwhelmed with all the negative energy and wanting to protect the vulnerable in her pack—the children. It was a horrible pattern.

Why did it feel so impossible?

I tried all the parenting advice again and again. I presented incentives, warned of consequences. I tried to level with him by having calm conversations on our mile-long walks home from school. How could we work better as a mommy and son team? "You mean *mom* and son team," he corrected me. He wasn't a baby anymore; I was MOM now. We would shake on it, hug it out, pinky swear. At bedtime, we would assert that the next morning would be different.

And then, it would not be different. He would wake up in a bad mood and I would be triggered.

One morning, I steeled myself and mentally repeated what my husband had kept saying to me: "De-escalate, de-escalate."

"I'm NOT eating this egg, it's disgusting! I don't like it like this, ewwww, you boiled it too long! Ew, no!"

De-escalate, de-escalate, I told myself. I kept my mouth shut. *I will not rise to this. I am the adult. I will not shout today.*

Then, out of seemingly nowhere, our dog started barking—at *me!* It was so surprising. What was she barking at? I hadn't shouted! I was deescalating!

And it hit me: My dog could sense my energy. My anger. It didn't matter that I wasn't shouting. That was purely external. Inside, the rage was still there.

The reason all the parenting techniques weren't working in these challenging moments was because I wasn't addressing the actual issue. The actual issue was within me, and it had started before I ever became a parent, possibly before I was even born.

*   *   *

Maya Angelou said, "Do the best you can until you know better. Then when you know better, do better."

Becoming a mother has brought so much to the surface—not only about traumatic experiences but also about my emotions, limitations, and needs—and with as many realizations as I have had, I often feel like I'm left with even more questions. The repair and communication that we parents are told to do these days was not something my parents did, and yet this—this truth-telling—is where healing begins.

In order to tell the truth, we first need to know and understand what the truth is. Acknowledging and accepting all the brokenness we hold within—through our memories, the stories we carry, our symptoms, our perceived failures—is also recognizing that we very well may have the exact abilities we need to mend our brokenness.

As Kelly Hoover Greenway reported in 2021 for *The Washington Post*, "[M]any experts think . . . that inherited trauma is our biology looking out for us, even if it may not appear that way at first. Experts said that studying inherited trauma is not meant to disempower or blame parents for things they cannot control. 'When we think about inheriting trauma, we think of something that is not good, but really what we're saying is that our bodies are resilient and trying to offset any potential traumas by allowing us to survive, and ultimately to thrive,' says Courtney Bolton, a Nashville-based child and family psychologist."[1]

This is what my anger was trying to teach me. My anger was demanding to be released from its unconscious dormancy so that it could help me heal, so that I could shatter the cycle. I didn't need to be ashamed or afraid of my anger; I needed to understand the truth and validity of it.

And Mark Wolynn, author of *It Didn't Start With You*, reminds us, "When a resolution isn't made in a family, the aspects of trauma can show up in later generations. Unconsciously we'll repeat a pattern and we'll share a similar unhappiness as our parents or grandparents until that trauma finally has a chance to heal."[2]

In order to break the cycle, Wolynn advises parents to "tell [your children] the terrible things that happened to you and whatever you know about what happened to your parents and your grandparents. They could be the unwitting recipients of painful feelings from the past. When you tell them what tragedies smolder in the family history, it can come as a great relief to them—especially if they make the connection that they've been carrying what belongs to you or to your parents or grandparents."[3]

On his website, Dr. Amen affirms this need to talk about what happened in the past: "Families can make resilience their new legacy by actively seeking to address the trauma. Building resilience through open and loving communication between generations is one of the best ways to loosen generational trauma's grip. Healing happens when family members speak up and work through any hurt, pain, or abuse from the past. If you are a parent, mental health experts suggest that you seek your own support and share your trauma openly with your children and possibly your grandchildren too. Tell them your story."[4]

Any belief that as a parent you're protecting your children by hiding parts of your history from them is misguided and ultimately very likely to be harmful. As Certified Parent Coach Meghan Leahy wrote in a 2017 piece for *The Washington Post*, "[T]he thing with kids in the midst of a crisis: They feel everything. The younger the children, the less they understand what they are feeling. But [they know] that something is up. . . . Unfortunately . . . kids assume that all the weird energy is about them. Children are focused on themselves—and that is how it is supposed to be."[5]

This means that when children are on the receiving end of a parent's trauma response, be it through physical abuse, emotional neglect, or uncontrolled rage, they will likely blame themselves. I know I did as a child. I kept trying to be different, to be better, so I could stop making my mom angry and depressed, so I could fix her. This eventually led to my internalizing and acting out her traumas. If only there had been moments of repair—if only I had been told, even occasionally, that it wasn't my fault or my responsibility—I believe it would have weakened the velocity of the cycle. I've learned so much about resilience and reparation as a parent myself: When we apologize and take accountability with our own children, not only do we free them from the burdens of our mistakes, we show them how they can handle their own.

Breaking the cycle is possible—and essential—whether it is a cycle deeply entrenched in the trauma of your ancestors or a cycle of a parent incapable of showing love. We *can* and *must* figure out a way to not repeat the mistakes of the past.

*   *   *

People had been right about me. I did have anger issues. It felt completely tied to my mom's anger. I was repeating what she had done to me—lashing out at my child over things that didn't require that level of reaction from me. I was acting at a ten when the situation required an authoritative and controlled three. Just like my mom had done when I made mistakes during piano practice. I felt overcome with heaviness that despite my best efforts and all the therapy I had been in, I was the same as her. I was repeating her mistakes.

But there was something about the inappropriateness of the rage that felt confusing. I didn't feel like it was accurate to just label myself as "an angry, fiery person." As I was understanding how I was repeating what had been done to me—unconsciously, automatically, as if I had been programmed to—I noticed another layer of my anger. Anger that my mother's abuse was still impacting me into adulthood, into my own parenthood. Wasn't it enough that I'd been through it all in the first place? I now had to figure out how to disengage from being just like her?

The all-encompassing, irrational rage—that wasn't mine. That was hers, that I had absorbed, that I was blindly perpetuating. But that quieter anger underneath, the one that was angry at my mom's anger—that WAS mine.

Realizing something this powerful is hard to process alone. When emotions are involved—your own, especially that have roots in childhood or your ancestral past—it's impossible to be your own objective observer. I write to organize my thoughts, or sometimes just to unburden myself from their weighty residency in my mind, but I'm often left trailing off . . . wondering okay, so now what? What do I do with this information?

For me, therapy has been an undeniable necessity. There is something about having a standing appointment with a trusted professional that keeps me anchored to the present moment. I can't call my therapist at will any time of day (I mean, I could, but he would probably have terminated our relationship?), which gives me time to steady myself. Having to wait until my session shows me that I can hold the heaviness of what I'm processing while being in my life, with my family, doing what I need to do. As painful as realizations and memories may feel, I've learned that they are not dangerous to me in the here and now. I am safe. I am an adult. I do not live with my mother anymore.

I told my therapist about my mother's internalized rage, how I was a textbook victim and perpetrator of generational trauma, and how angry and ashamed I felt. He helped me understand the part of my rage that was, actually, righteous. My rage was from the little me who was hit, berated, ignored, and emotionally abandoned by the one person in the world who I was supposed to be able to count on the most. I had been hit with waves of *sadness* when I first became a mother and started realizing that I, as a child, had not received all the motherly things I endeavored to do for my child. But becoming acquainted with my childhood *rage* was a new depth.

As I thought about my younger self, I worked to absolve myself of the shame around being labeled as fiery, having a short fuse, and having anger issues. Of course I had anger issues. My mom beat me because I made mistakes in piano or because she thought I looked at her a certain way that she disapproved of. I had every right to feel angry about being treated like I was worthless. I had every right to feel angry that nobody stood up for me, asked me if I was okay. I do have a few memories of my dad walking into some of these beatings, and stopping my mom, ushering her away as she was hyperventilating, shrieking in a rage, calling me hurtful names in Korean, the true meanings of which I continue to try to understand as there is no precise English translation.

I always felt grateful for the times that he stopped it, but how I wish that he had come back to talk to me, to tell me that what had happened was not okay, to tell me that he would keep me safe. As my parent, he should have. And yet I understand why he didn't, why he couldn't. I don't think he knew the impact he could have had by simply acknowledging my fear. Maybe I could have at least been saved from blaming myself or questioning my own intuition. I don't blame him; we all come from such intergenerational brokenness.

But me—I am committed to being a cycle breaker. This madness stops with me. I may have endured a lot, but I have also been luckier than my parents in many ways because I was born into a culture that gave me a glimpse of a different way of dealing with difficult emotions, even if, as a woman of color, I would have to fight to be supported and heard. My mom's trauma tried to pull me into its orbit—sometimes by literally pulling me through the house by my hair—but I fought to survive. I steadied my gaze on an exit plan. I got help when I felt like I was drowning in a depression and anxiety that felt familiar to my mother's. I am making different choices.

In one of my first therapy sessions, I had fearfully asked, "Do you think I am going to end up like her? I mean, I have her genes."

My therapist answered, "You are not your mother. You share *some* genes, but you have your own mind, your own awareness. You can make your own choices. You're already on a different path to hers because you're here."

This was the most important life raft I was ever thrown.

*   *   *

What my therapist helped me understand during our sessions is echoed by therapist Sahaj Kaur Kohli. In our interview, she explained, "When we change the way that we react, respond, communicate, show up in a relationship, when we know how to better regulate and ground ourselves, when we learn those skills, even if no one else in our family is going to therapy, we change things. I am showing up in my family system differently. I am learning how to handle the guilt differently, to get less defensive around my parents, to see things from new perspectives. I am no longer on edge. I am no longer easy to anger. I am no longer avoidant. I am no longer struggling with how to share my feelings. I'm more grounded and because I'm showing up differently just by default, the people around me show up differently because relationships are a two-way street. We feed off of each other's energies, tools, skills, and capacities in all relationships. That's why you have some relationships where it feels like you're doing more work, and you have some relationships where it feels more equal, or you have some relationships where you're just stuck in the cycle of conflict that looks the same every day because you're feeding off of each other.

"And so when you do the work, when I do the work and we show up differently, by default, the relationship is going to look different. And when we change, the relationship changes and therefore the other person changes. And I'm not saying it's just like macro growth progress, but the progress maybe looks like a baby step in the right direction, which is change, which is healing.

"When you're a more healed version of yourself, you're allowing people to show up as a different version of themselves too. I think just showing up differently has ripple effects to how other people show up. And then we are modeling and teaching some of those skills now. When you are more healed version of yourself and you are a parent, you are going to be healing that next generation by just showing up more healed.

"That's what it means to address intergenerational trauma and break those cycles. There's that literal sense of doing things differently than our parents did. And then there's showing up differently and letting the relationship evolve, which is a form of healing."

Kohli's framing is ultimately so empowering. We don't need the people we are in relationship with, with whom we share an inheritance of generational trauma, to go to therapy or to do anything else. We don't need to convince anyone else that they need to change. We don't even need anyone else to validate our suffering or our healing. Simply by us doing the work and showing up differently—showing up as a more healed version of ourselves—we necessarily change the dynamics we have with others. We direct the cycles of trauma. We guide our fates.

Notice, also, that Kohli speaks about healing as a process rather than an end goal. The work is in becoming a *more* healed version of ourselves, not a completely healed, perfect version of ourselves. I think this is such an important reminder especially in this cancel culture society that is so quick to call out mistakes and demand the impossibility of moral perfection. We are human beings, not AI. Even as we heal, process, and learn, there will be times that we aren't able to apply what we know. This doesn't mean that we are failing; it just means that we are constantly in the process of evolving.

*   *   *

Less than a month before my daughter's due date, I was at one of the many prenatal appointments that really ramp up in those last weeks, especially if you're of "advanced maternal age." My OBGYN asked me how I was feeling, and I answered honestly that I felt good and that I was also aware that postpartum darkness could be coming for me again. It occurred to me that we had never discussed my postpartum mental health after my son—I'd had him in London, after all. My doctor looked surprised and immediately pulled out his prescription pad.

"We should have started you on this six weeks before your due date, but you can still start now."

"Oh, but I never took an anti-depressant," I told him.

"That doesn't matter. It can still help to take it proactively. My sister had postpartum depression with her first baby, but she took medication at the end of her second pregnancy—she felt amazing! She had no postpartum issues!"

"That's really great for her, and I know medication can really help, but it's complicated for me. I'd like to ask my therapist before taking any prescription, since I've been seeing him for many years now."

While I know my OBGYN was coming from a place of care and concern, I also couldn't help but feel that he was jumping to medication without any psychological analysis or support, which was outside of his specialty. He was my doctor to help me have a safe and healthy pregnancy and delivery; he wasn't a therapist or psychiatrist. I am grateful that I had the self-knowing and confidence to advocate for myself to be able to set boundaries.

Because as it turns out—I did not have postpartum depression following the birth of my daughter. By the time I was pregnant with her, everyone close to me in my life knew that I had struggled badly after my son. And so I had many, many loved ones checking in on me. I think that fact alone—the fact that I was not alone—was healing in and of itself. I didn't have to pretend, I didn't have to hide, I didn't have to be ashamed.

I remember telling a friend on a phone call, "I keep waiting for the depression to come, like a monster about to jump out and scare me, but there's been nothing. I'm starting to think maybe I'm free?"

Something in my psychology and physiology had indeed evolved, enabling me to have a more easeful experience during the newborn season the second time around. The work of understanding trauma, of shattering cycles—it sets us all free.

Accepting the rage that exists within me has weakened its stronghold on my reactivity when I am triggered. I am no longer programmed to always skyrocket to a ten.

The first time I was able to keep my rage separate from a stressful moment, it felt nothing short of a miracle. My son had woken up grumpy, complaining about his clothes and his breakfast. Instead of repeating the horrible pattern I had gotten us stuck in, I was able to respond appropriately as a level-headed, loving parent. The rage just wasn't there in that moment—I was even actively searching for it! There was no barking from the dog. And as a result, instead of the usual shouting back and forth, my son almost instantly became accountable: "Oh sorry, Mom, that was rude."

It sounds too good to be true, doesn't it? But like a baby that cries incessantly when he wants to be picked up and stops crying as soon as he is cuddled, once I acknowledged and softened around my rage, its insistent intensity started to extinguish. Once I placed my childhood rage where it belonged—in the past—it was as if it no longer felt the need to plow into every hard moment to make itself known.

The grooves of old patterning are still there. I don't know that they will ever be erased completely. I still lose my temper and yell; it never helps. But when I do, I catch myself more quickly, and I always apologize and repair: "I'm sorry I yelled. I am the adult, I am the parent. I am the one that needs to stay calm. Let's work together to find a solution for this issue."

By identifying emotions and memories and by recognizing what happened to me and affirming that what happened was not okay, it was like I put up a Do Not Enter sign on the well-traveled route and showed myself a new, alternate route. I don't have to be controlled by my rage, my pain, my past. I don't have to repeat cycles of trauma. I can set myself—and therefore my children—free.

As Kohli reminds us, "Being a cycle breaker can be really painful. It can be really hard to work on disrupting patterns and recognizing what might need to be broken. But it's also about being present during your experiences and recognizing what my lineage is that is carrying me forward with strength and resilience and adaptability. I think that that's such a beautiful way to reframe generational trauma."

I believe mothers are the best equipped to be cycle breakers because we are always holding the nuance of the both / and. We intimately live the daily dichotomy of motherhood. At once wanting the day's asks and chores to be over and done with while also wishing time would move just a bit slower. Being relieved that the days of endless diaper changes and feedings are behind us while desperately missing those tiny toes, those first words, the toddling first steps, that newborn smell. The weight of worry alongside the greatest, purest love we could ever imagine—we hold it all in our very mothering.

None of this is work for the weary but here's the thing: we got this. As mothers, we exist with our hearts outside of our bodies. We created and sustained life with our literal cells. We are always in the pursuit of growing our souls and we understand that the children are always ours, every single one of them, all over the globe. (I am ever grateful to Grace Lee Boggs and James Baldwin for the endless literary breadcrumbs they left behind, always guiding us back to our humanity.)

It is for each and every child, from those that are lucky enough to be tucked safe and sound in their own homes to those displaced in unimaginable conditions around the world, that we mothers commit to healing, to shattering cycles and systems of hierarchy, and to building enduring connections and communities.

Conclusion

I have often heard that writing a book is a birthing process. A book, while being written, is most certainly a living, evolving entity that ultimately finds permanence in its eventual printing and publishing. I have changed so much from the inception of *Mom, Unfiltered*; we—the book and I—have changed together.

My case for prioritizing the mental health of mothers as an essential part of both the mother and her children's well-being remains unchanged. If anything, the many hours of conversations and research as well as my ongoing and deepening relationships with my beloved son and daughter have only convinced me of the power of a mother's healing.

I have tried to connect a lot of dots in this book and I recognize that it's impossible for me to touch upon all the issues that are critical to maternal mental health. I have undoubtedly left gaps in the tapestry; I hope other mothers will weave in their own stories of healing.

There is so much more we can learn about each other, particularly about people with different backgrounds and identities. I couldn't believe how uninformed I was on the statistics pertaining to Black pregnant birthing people and the ongoing dehumanization of our Indigenous mothers and children. I have so much more to learn but this much is clear: we must show up and speak up for each other. For guidance, we can look to fellow mothers and especially to midwives like Robina Khalid, doulas like Ashley Simpo, and our elders. I am so excited that the world of psychotherapy is evolving with radical femmes such as Candice Rose Valenzuela, Sahaj Kaur Kohli, Alisha Bennett, Lena Derhally, and Melissa Bada-Devers. I believe that we can get closer to the roots of sacred practices with educators like Lindsey Guttilla, Joon Ae Haworth-Kaufka, and Roberta Sam. I am grateful for the holistic lenses of healthcare professionals such as Sarah Chung, Pyravin Abbasova, Laura Iu, and Amber Bloom.

I believe we are all here to do our part. I believe we are meant to be here, during this time of calamity, chaos, and crisis. Great Ones that have come before us, from Heraclitus to the Buddha, have said that change is the only constant in life. How can we be a part of the change that brings us home to each other? What can we change within ourselves and in our ancestral lineages to move collectively toward healing?

Motherhood continues to surprise me constantly. My daughter snuck into her closet and chopped off chunks of her hair the other day. It was the first time I've ever experienced this happening! My son recently told me, so casually, that I am known among his classmates as one of the nice and chill moms. I tried, in vain, to hide my absolute exuberance upon hearing this.

Every single day, I think about the children who are suffering around the world. I believe that we are all inextricably connected to each other, at least on a soul level, and so with all my heart, I hope that the love I have and hold for my children somehow translates, if only in some tiny way, to those who deserve so much—so unbelievably much—better. At the very least, may it mean something for our collective humanity that I, along with my husband, am raising our children to be in their truth. May we all shepherd our children to be stewards of justice, empathy, and love.

Notes

Chapter 1

1 The American College of Obstetricians and Gynecologists, "How Your Fetus Grows During Pregnancy,"
https://www.acog.org/womens-health/faqs/how-your-fetus-grows-during
-pregnancy (21 May 2025).

2 National Health Service, "My Waters Have Broken and I'm Not Having Contractions," https://www.buckshealthcare.nhs.uk/birthchoices/pifs/my
-waters-have-broken-and-i-am-not-having-contractions/ (9 February 2025)

3 National Institute of Mental Health, "Coping With Traumatic Events."
https://www.nimh.nih.gov/health/topics/coping-with-traumatic-events (May 2024)

4 National Institute of Mental Health, "Perinatal Depression," https://www
.nimh.nih.gov/health/publications/perinatal-depression (2023)

5 National Health Service, "Caring for Your Wound After Having a Caesarean Section," https://www.mkuh.nhs.uk/patient-information-leaflet/caring-for
-your-wound-after-having-a-caesarean-section

Chapter 2

1 National Childbirth Trust, "Traumatic Birth and Post-Traumatic Stress,"
https://www.mkuh.nhs.uk/patient-information-leaflet/caring-for-your
-wound-after-having-a-caesarean-section (July 2022)

2 Dr. Uché Blackstock, Legacy: A Black Physician Reckons with Racism in Medicine, page 29 (2024)

3 Dr. Uché Blackstock, Legacy: A Black Physician Reckons with Racism in Medicine, page 150 (2024)

4 Dr. Uché Blackstock, Legacy: A Black Physician Reckons with Racism in Medicine, page 152 (2024)

5 Dr. Uché Blackstock, Legacy: A Black Physician Reckons with Racism in Medicine, page 159 (2024)

6 The McGill Office for Science and Society, "40 Years of Human Experimentation in America: The Tuskegee Study," https://www.mcgill.ca /oss/article/history/40-years-human-experimentation-america-tuskegee -study (25 January 2019)

7 The McGill Office for Science and Society, "40 Years of Human Experimentation in America: The Tuskegee Study," https://www.mcgill.ca /oss/article/history/40-years-human-experimentation-america-tuskegee -study (25 January 2019)

8 The Lancet, Bill Bynum, "Discarded Diagnoses," https://www.thelancet.com /journals/lancet/article/PIIS0140-6736(05)74468-8/abstract (4 November 2000)

9 The McGill Office for Science and Society, Ada McVean B.Sc., "40 Years of Human Experimentation in America: The Tuskegee Study," https://www .mcgill.ca/oss/article/history/40-years-human-experimentation-america -tuskegee-study (25 January 2019)

10 ELLE, Serena Williams, "How Serena Williams Saved Her Own Life," https://www.elle.com/life-love/a39586444/how-serena-williams-saved-her -own-life/ (5 April 2022)

11 ELLE, Serena Williams, "How Serena Williams Saved Her Own Life," https://www.elle.com/life-love/a39586444/how-serena-williams-saved-her -own-life/ (5 April 2022)

12 ELLE, Serena Williams, "How Serena Williams Saved Her Own Life," https://www.elle.com/life-love/a39586444/how-serena-williams-saved-her -own-life/ (5 April 2022)

13 Dr. Uché Blackstock, Legacy: A Black Physician Reckons with Racism in Medicine, page 154 (2024)

14 npr, Shankar Vedantam et al, "Remembering Anarcha, Lucy, and Betsey: The Mothers of Modern Gynecology," https://www.npr.org/2017/02/07

/513764158/remembering-anarcha-lucy-and-betsey-the-mothers-of
-modern-gynecology (7 February 2017)

15 npr, Hidden Brain Podcast, Shankar Vedantam et al, "Remembering Anarcha, Lucy, and Betsey: The Mothers of Modern Gynecology," https:// www.npr.org/2017/02/07/513764158/remembering-anarcha-lucy-and -betsey-the-mothers-of-modern-gynecology (7 February 2017)

16 UCLA Women's Law Journal, "The Norplant Solution: Norplant and the Control of African-American Motherhood," https://escholarship.org/uc/ item/9861n279 (1995)

17 In Our Own Voice: National Black Women's Reproductive Justice Agenda, "Reimagining Policy: In Pursuit of Black Reproductive Justice," https:// blackrj.org/wp-content/uploads/2023/06/RJPolicyAgenda2023.pdf (2023)

18 Rosemary Campbell Stephens, "Masterclass: Moving from ethnic minority to Global Majority," https://rosemarycampbellstephens.com/service-post/ keynotes-on-the-global-majority-mindset/

19 Mayo Clinic, "COVID-19 infections by race: What's behind the health disparities?" https://www.mayoclinic.org/diseases-conditions/coronavirus/ expert-answers/coronavirus-infection-by-race/faq-20488802 (6 July 2024)

20 University of College London, "Lessons must be learnt from Covid-19's unequal impact on minority groups," https://www.ucl.ac.uk/news/2023/jul /lessons-must-be-learnt-covid-19s-unequal-impact-minority-groups (27 July 2023)

21 March of Dimes, "Maternal death and pregnancy-related death," https:// www.marchofdimes.org/find-support/topics/miscarriage-loss-grief/ maternal-death-and-pregnancy-related-death (April 2024)

Chapter 4

1 The Canadian Journal of Psychiatry, John J. Sigal, Ph.D. and Vivian Rakoff, M.D., "Concentration Camp Survival: A Pilot Study of Effects on the Second Generation," https://journals.sagepub.com/doi/abs/10.1177 /070674377101600503 (October 1971)

2 Psychology Today, Elizabeth Dixon, LISW-CP, "Breaking the Chains of Generational Trauma," https://www.psychologytoday.com/us/blog/the

-flourishing-family/202107/breaking-the-chains-generational-trauma (3 July 2021)

3 health, Claire Gillespie, "What Is Generational Trauma?" https://www .health.com/condition/ptsd/generational-trauma (13 March 2025)

4 health, Claire Gillespie, "What Is Generational Trauma?" https://www .health.com/condition/ptsd/generational-trauma (13 March 2025)

5 Amen Clinics, "Can You Stop the Cycle of Generational Trauma?" https:// www.amenclinics.com/blog/can-you-stop-the-cycle-of-generational-trauma (19 April 2022)

6 American Psychological Association, Tori DeAngelis, "The legacy of trauma," https://www.apa.org/monitor/2019/02/legacy-trauma (February 2019)

7 American Psychological Association, Tori DeAngelis, "The legacy of trauma," https://www.apa.org/monitor/2019/02/legacy-trauma (February 2019)

8 Journal of Clinical Nursing, Sophie Isobel, "Preventing intergenerational trauma transmission: A critical interpretive synthesis," https://onlinelibrary .wiley.com/doi/10.1111/jocn.14735 (16 December 2018)

9 Gerald Litwack, Human Biochemistry, page 287 (2021)

10 Mark Wolynn, It Didn't Start With You: How Inherited Family Trauma Shapes Who We Are and How to End the Cycle, page 29 (2016)

11 On Being with Krista Tippett podcast, "Rachel Yehuda: How Trauam and Resilience Cross Generations," https://onbeing.org/programs/rachel-yehuda -how-trauma-and-resilience-cross-generations-nov2017/ (30 July 2015)

12 The Korea Times, Lee Hyo-jin, "History of OPCON transfer talks between South Korea, US," https://www.koreatimes.co.kr/southkorea/defense /20250305/history-of-opcon-transfer-negotiations-between-south-korea-us (5 March 2025)

13 U.S. Department of Defense, "Defense Vision of the U.S.-ROK Alliance," https://www.defense.gov/News/Releases/Release/Article/3586528/defense -vision-of-the-us-rok-alliance/ (13 November 2023)

Chapter 5

1 The Oxford Review, "Hyperindividualism – Definition and Explanation," https://oxford-review.com/the-oxford-review-dei-diversity-equity-and-inclusion-dictionary/hyperindividualism-definition-and-explanation/

2 Worldwide Independent Network of Market Research, "Women's Safety Emerges as a Global Concern," https://winmr.com/womens-safety-emerges-as-a-global-concern/ (22 March 2024)

3 USA FACTS, "How many moms are in the labor force?" https://usafacts.org/articles/how-many-mothers-are-in-the-labor-force/ (29 December 2023)

4 UNICEF, "How many babies are born a year?" https://data.unicef.org/how-many/how-many-babies-are-born-a-year/ 2024

5 La Leche League GB, Emma Taylor, "Life with a new baby across the world," https://laleche.org.uk/life-with-a-new-baby-across-the-world/

6 The New York Times, Lauretta Charlton, "For New Moms in Seoul, 3 Weeks of Pampering and Sleep at a Joriwon," https://www.nytimes.com/2024/01/28/world/asia/south-korea-joriwon-postpartum-care.html (28 January 2024)

7 The New York Times, Lauretta Charlton, "For New Moms in Seoul, 3 Weeks of Pampering and Sleep at a Joriwon," https://www.nytimes.com/2024/01/28/world/asia/south-korea-joriwon-postpartum-care.html (28 January 2024)

8 Harvard, "Loneliness in America: How the Pandemic Has Deepened an Epidemic of Loneliness and What We Can Do About It," https://mcc.gse.harvard.edu/reports/loneliness-in-america (February 2021)

9 Britannica, "nuclear family," https://www.britannica.com/topic/nuclear-family (25 April 2025)

10 National Library of Medicine, Paulo Andrade Lotufo, "Why we should contain the 'medical-industrial-media complex," https://pmc.ncbi.nlm.nih.gov/articles/PMC11115344/ (1 March 2004)

11 American Hospital Association, "Fast Facs on U.S. Hospitals, 2025," https://www.aha.org/statistics/fast-facts-us-hospitals (January 2025)

Chapter 6

1 The American College of Obstetricians and Gynecologists, "Optimizing Postpartum Care," https://www.acog.org/-/media/project/acog/acogorg/clinical/files/committee-opinion/articles/2018/05/optimizing-postpartum-care.pdf (5 May 2018)

2 The American College of Obstetricians and Gynecologists, Dr. Diana Ramos, "What to Expect at a Postpartum Checkup – And Why the Visit Matters," https://www.acog.org/womens-health/experts-and-stories/the-latest/what-to-expect-at-a-postpartum-checkup-and-why-the-visit-matters (February 2024)

3 The American College of Obstetricians and Gynecologists, "Optimizing Postpartum Care," https://www.acog.org/-/media/project/acog/acogorg/clinical/files/committee-opinion/articles/2018/05/optimizing-postpartum-care.pdf (5 May 2018)

4 babycenter, Cassie Shortsleeve, "Postpartum care overlooksmoms, prioritizing only babies' needs: Survey," https://www.babycenter.com/baby/postpartum-health/postpartum-care-maternal-health-support-report_41001478 (17 October 2023)

5 Acta Psychologica, "How are mothers negatively affected and supported by following parenting-related Instagram profiles? A mixed-methods study," https://www.sciencedirect.com/science/article/pii/S0001691822001081?ref=pdf_download&fr=RR-2&rr=7ebf5a042c0e1889 (July 2022)

6 AMA Journal of Ethics, Mitzi M. Waltz, phD, "Mothers and Autism: The Evolution of a Discourse of Blame," https://journalofethics.ama-assn.org/article/mothers-and-autism-evolution-discourse-blame/2015-04 (April 2015)

7 PYMNTS, "New Reality Check: The Paycheck-to-Paycheck Report," https://www.pymnts.com/study/reality-check-paycheck-to-paycheck-revolving-debt-financing-credit-scores/ (December 2023)

8 The New York Times, Jessica Grose, "Why Are Momfluencers So Good at Worming Their Way Into Your Brain?" https://www.nytimes.com/2022/11/22/opinion/influencers-moms-parenting.html (22 November 2022)

Chapter 7

1 CDC, "Vital Signs: Postpartum Depressive Symptoms and Proivder Discussion About Perinatal Depression – United States, 2018," https://www.cdc.gov/mmwr/volumes/69/wr/mm6919a2.htm (15 May 2020)

2 American Psychological Association, Luona Lin, MPP, "How diverse is the psychology workforce?" https://www.apa.org/monitor/2018/02/datapoint (February 2018)

3 CDC, "Births Rose for the First Time in Seven Years in 2021," https://www.cdc.gov/nchs/pressroom/nchs_press_releases/2022/20220524.htm (24 May 2022)

4 UNICEF, "Nearly 386,000 children will be born worldwide on New Year's Day, says UNICEF," https://www.unicef.org/press-releases/nearly-386000-children-will-be-born-worldwide-new-years-day-says-unicef (1 January 2018)

5 Michigan Medicine, "A third of new moms had postpartum depression during early COVID," https://www.michiganmedicine.org/health-lab/third-new-moms-had-postpartum-depression-during-early-covid (23 March 2022)

6 PostpartumDepression.org, "Postpartum Depression Statistics," https://www.postpartumdepression.org/postpartum-depression/

7 Postpartum Progress, Katherine Stone, "How Many Women Get Postpartum Depression? The Statistics on PPD," https://postpartumprogress.com/how-many-women-get-postpartum-depression-the-statistics-on-ppd

8 Postpartum Progress, Katherine Stone, "How Many Women Get Postpartum Depression? The Statistics on PPD," https://postpartumprogress.com/how-many-women-get-postpartum-depression-the-statistics-on-ppd

9 Maternal Mental Health Leadership Alliance, "Maternal Mental Health Conditions: The Most Common Complication of Pregnancy and Parenting," https://www.mmhla.org/articles/maternal-mental-health-conditions-the-most-common-complication-of-pregnancy-and-parenting (9 May 2024)

10 PostpartumDepression.org, "Postpartum Depression Statistics," https://www.postpartumdepression.org/resources/statistics/

11 PostpartumDepression.org, "Postpartum Depression Statistics," https://www.postpartumdepression.org/resources/statistics/

12　Scientific American, Dana G. Smith, "An Entirely New Type of Antidepressant Targets Postpartum Depression," https://www.scientificamerican.com/article/an-entirely-new-type-of-antidepressant-targets-postpartum-depression/ (15 August 2018)

13　National Library of Medicine, "Postpartum depression," https://pmc.ncbi.nlm.nih.gov/articles/PMC3918890/

14　National Library of Medicine, "Racial and Ethnic Disparities in Postpartum Depression Care Among Low-Income Women," https://pmc.ncbi.nlm.nih.gov/articles/PMC3733216/

15　National Alliance on Mental Illness, "Medicaid Coverage for Maternal Mental Health," https://www.nami.org/Advocacy/Policy-Priorities/Improving-Health/Medicaid-Coverage-for-Maternal-Mental-Health/

16　The American College of Obstetricians and Gynecologists, "Optimizing Postpartum Care," https://www.acog.org/clinical/clinical-guidance/committee-opinion/articles/2018/05/optimizing-postpartum-care (May 2018)

17　The New York Times, Yara M. Asi, "The Trauma Experienced in Gaza Is Beyond PTSD," https://www.nytimes.com/2024/02/22/opinion/gaza-palestinians-mental-health.html (22 February 2024)

Chapter 8

1　Tricycle, Tina Fossella, "Human Nature, Buddha Nature," https://tricycle.org/magazine/human-nature-buddha-nature/ (Spring 2011)

2　Journal of Spirituality in Mental Health, Gabriela Picciotto, "A phenomenology of spiritual bypass: Causes, consequences, and implications," https://www.tandfonline.com/doi/full/10.1080/19349637.2017.1417756?src=recsys (11 October 2017)

3　Yoga Alliance, "First of Its Kind Global Study of Yoga Reveals Stress Management and Mental Health Are Driving Growing Interest and Participation, Yet Many Underserved," https://blog.yogaalliance.org/2023/11/15/press-release-yoga-in-the-world-research-study/ (15 November 2023)

4　Yoga Alliance, "First of Its Kind Global Study of Yoga Reveals Stress Management and Mental Health Are Driving Growing Interest and

Participation, Yet Many Underserved," https://blog.yogaalliance.org/2023/11/15/press-release-yoga-in-the-world-research-study/ (15 November 2023)

5 Yoga Alliance, "First of Its Kind Global Study of Yoga Reveals Stress Management and Mental Health Are Driving Growing Interest and Participation, Yet Many Underserved," https://blog.yogaalliance.org/2023/11/15/press-release-yoga-in-the-world-research-study/ (15 November 2023)

6 Yoga Alliance, "First of Its Kind Global Study of Yoga Reveals Stress Management and Mental Health Are Driving Growing Interest and Participation, Yet Many Underserved," https://blog.yogaalliance.org/2023/11/15/press-release-yoga-in-the-world-research-study/ (15 November 2023)

7 Yoga Alliance, "First of Its Kind Global Study of Yoga Reveals Stress Management and Mental Health Are Driving Growing Interest and Participation, Yet Many Underserved," https://blog.yogaalliance.org/2023/11/15/press-release-yoga-in-the-world-research-study/ (15 November 2023)

8 Yoga Alliance, "First of Its Kind Global Study of Yoga Reveals Stress Management and Mental Health Are Driving Growing Interest and Participation, Yet Many Underserved," https://blog.yogaalliance.org/2023/11/15/press-release-yoga-in-the-world-research-study/ (15 November 2023)

9 Yoga Alliance, "First of Its Kind Global Study of Yoga Reveals Stress Management and Mental Health Are Driving Growing Interest and Participation, Yet Many Underserved," https://blog.yogaalliance.org/2023/11/15/press-release-yoga-in-the-world-research-study/ (15 November 2023)

Chapter 9

1 GOV.UK, "Regional Ethnic Diversity," https://www.ethnicity-facts-figures.service.gov.uk/uk-population-by-ethnicity/national-and-regional-populations/regional-ethnic-diversity/latest/#main-facts-and-figures (22 December 2022)

2 Slate, Jordan Weissmann, "Senator Says Legalizing Interracial Marriage Was a Mistake, Backtracks Unconvincingly," https://slate.com/news-and-politics/2022/03/republican-sen-mike-braun-says-supreme-court-should-not-have-struck-down-state-laws-banning-interracial-marriage-then-backtracks-unconvincingly.html (22 March 2022)

Chapter 10

1 The Washington Post, Kelly Hoover Greenway, "Why Understanding Inherited Trauma is Critical, and What it Means for Our Kids," https://www .washingtonpost.com/lifestyle/2021/07/19/inherited-trauma-family-kids/ (19 July 2021)

2 Wellness + Wisdom, "Mark Wolynn," https://wellnessforce.com/mark -wolynn-how-to-heal-generational-trauma/

3 Wellness + Wisdom, "Mark Wolynn," https://wellnessforce.com/mark -wolynn-how-to-heal-generational-trauma/

4 Amen Clinics, "Can You Stop the Cycle of Generational Trauma?" https:// www.amenclinics.com/blog/can-you-stop-the-cycle-of-generational-trauma/ (19 April 2022)

5 The Washington Post, Meghan Leahy, "How to explain a family trauma to a 7-year-old? Consider telling her the truth." https://www.washingtonpost.com /lifestyle/on-parenting/our-7-year-old-knows-something-is-up-how-do-we -tell-her-that-her-older-sister-was-sexually-assaulted/2017/10/10/473c897a -aa80-11e7-b3aa-c0e2e1d41e38_story.html (11 October 2017)

Index

About the Author

Leah Kim started teaching yoga in 2005 after studying English, Korean, and Economics at UCLA. As Nike's Global Yoga Ambassador for a decade, she led classes, events, and trainings all over the world, from local yoga studios to Apple Headquarters. When Leah was pregnant with her first child, she designed and filmed a pregnancy yoga series and thought she would be an example of how a new mother can bounce back and have it all. Instead, she found herself in a prolonged period of postpartum depression.

Leah is a storyteller with a uniquely nuanced understanding of mental health and the intersection of motherhood, trauma, and racial oppression. She writes because she feels compelled to support others in order to collectively break cycles and move toward freedom. She is the host of *Voices on the Side* and the co-host of *Cha*, podcasts which center the stories of marginalized identities.

Leah lives with her husband, two children, and Goldendoodle in New York City.